Fries, Thighs, and Lies

The Girlfriend's Guide to Getting the Skinny on Fat

DEBORAH ARNESON,
B.S., M.S., L.C.N.

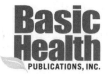
Basic Health
PUBLICATIONS, INC.

The information contained in this book is based upon the research and personal and professional experiences of the author. It is not intended as a substitute for consulting with your physician or other healthcare provider. Any attempt to diagnose and treat an illness should be done under the direction of a healthcare professional.

The publisher does not advocate the use of any particular healthcare protocol but believes the information in this book should be available to the public. The publisher and author are not responsible for any adverse effects or consequences resulting from the use of the suggestions, preparations, or procedures discussed in this book. Should the reader have any questions concerning the appropriateness of any procedures or preparation mentioned, the author and the publisher strongly suggest consulting a professional healthcare advisor.

Basic Health Publications, Inc.
28812 Top of the World Drive
Laguna Beach, CA 92651
949-715-7327 • www.basichealthpub.com

Library of Congress Cataloging-in-Publication Data

Arneson, Deborah.
    Fries, thighs, and lies : the girlfriend's guide to getting the skinny on fat /
Deborah Arneson.
      p. cm.
    ISBN-13: 978-1-59120-194-6
    ISBN-10: 1-59120-194-2
  1. Weight loss—Popular works. 2. Women—Health and hygiene—Popular
works. I. Title.

    RM222.2.A74   2007
    613.2'5—dc22
                                 2006100735

Editor: Roberta W. Waddell • Copyeditor: Kristen Jennings
Book design and typesetting: Gary A. Rosenberg • Cover design: Mike Stromberg

Printed in the United States of America

10   9   8   7   6   5   4   3   2   1

Contents

I dedicate this book to Mike Tyler,
my dear friend and an extraordinary visionary
who saw the depth of my knowledge
and believed in my ability to help so many.

Acknowledgments

I wish to thank Jeremiah Padula, the wind beneath my wings, who believed in me, and who convinced me I could do anything and be the very best at whatever I chose to do. I chose to believe.

I would especially like to acknowledge as an inspiration my father, Richard Arneson, who wouldn't let me quit, and who, in his quiet, observing way, hoisted me a number of life rafts, helping to keep my business afloat.

A special acknowledgment to my dear friend Sid Luckman, human being extraordinaire, my business and life mentor who always told me to hold my head high, put my best foot forward, and strut like a peacock. This was an extraordinary man who left our planet far too soon.

And to Kristi Oleson, my sister of the heart. Unflappable, beyond generous, beautiful to behold, and of undaunted spirit, she keeps my life surrounded by beauty with her creativity and design talents.

A warm heartfelt thank you to Barbara Bell, Mary Beth Shea, John Wagner, Doug Kaulas, and Charlene Gorzela, who have supported all my efforts to bring health to so many.

Thanks also to my two daughters, Christina and Susanna, as well as Susanna's husband, Doug, who all continue to support me over and over again in a million different ways. Their love has kept me whole and sane.

My heartfelt appreciation to my publisher, Norman Goldfind, for believing in my concept and moving my book from a dream to a reality; to Carolyn

Schwarzkopf, my precious assistant, who provided endless hours, endless attention to details, and endless caring; and to Bobby Waddell, my patient editor, who painstakingly guided me through the birthing process.

A sweet thank you to my thousands of clients, who have gifted me with their faith and trust. They have been my true teachers, bearing the seeds that have ripened into the fruit of all that I have learned from them in their personal quests for health and healing.

My deepest and most heartfelt appreciation and thank you to Mike Tyler, my dear friend and the wisest man I've met on this planet. Mike, without you none of this would have ever come to be. Thank you for gently coddling and convincing me for years *to just write the book—step out of my box and fly*. Your kindness, your humor, your heart, and your editing gifts are my blessing. Truly, without you this book would not be, my earthly angel man.

Preface

Damn, look at my behind! I eat fat-free cookies, drink diet soda . . .
and I've still got excess fat. Why is this fat on MY body?
What IS excess fat anyway?

*S*ound like a conversation you've had? Do you get motion sickness just thinking about walking down the street? Jiggle, jiggle? Wiggle, wiggle? Does your back fat fit into a C-cup? Girl, you and I need to talk.

Let me answer the *fat* question first. Fat is an assemblage of natural esters of glycerol combined with organic compounds consisting of a hydrocarbon chain plus . . . yadda, yadda, yadda. Who cares? To you, fat is buttery and creamy and delicious—except when it's ham-hocked on the back of your arms, weenie-rolled around your waist, or dimpled-up on your butt.

Many of you have been there. It's like having a rear end with its own zip code, which is one of the reasons I have spent more than two decades as a successful nutritionist counseling people. During that time, one thing I have learned for sure is that most people don't really care what a trans-fatty acid is, or whether or not white rice has a higher glycemic index than a Snickers bar. When it comes to weight control and fat loss, most people just care about what's easy to do, not what they should know, or what makes sense. That's why I wrote this book, to show you how to lose the weight called body fat.

But let me be up front about something. This is *not* a diet book. It's *not* a nutrition book, either. Surprised? Here's the good news: You won't be scanning pages with loads of serving charts, calorie tables (okay, maybe a couple of formulas here and there), or all that other stuff in all the other diet books you've bought and *never* read. Why write a big fat book about being thin? If it really is as easy as *Exercise, move it to lose it, and just eat right,* then you don't need 500 pages to explain that to you, right? I'm thinking no more than 200 pages.

What I *will* offer is some sit-on-your-grandma's-lap common sense about the relationship that's going on between your mind and your mouth; and girlfriend, you and I both know that can be a toxic love affair at times. So, take a look at how you can walk away from this dysfunctional relationship *forever.* That's right. Here's your new atti-TUNE: "Hit the road fat, and don't you come back, no more, no more, no more, no more . . . "

Put on your ruby slippers, Dorothy. Time to conquer your fear of fries, say *bye-bye* to thunder thighs, and reconcile all the lies that have led you to: *Lycra and diets and spare tires, oh my! Lycra and diets and spare tires, oh my!*

Deborah Arneson, B.S., M.S.
Licensed Clinical Nutritionist

Get Real

Remember that night, how he gazed into your eyes
from his supersized plate of golden French fries?
And as you gobbled up his lies, he headed straight for your thighs.
That's just Fat being FAT, and he'll always be like that.
It starts with the pinch and the grab.
Then he leaves you holding the flab.

*P*eople, knowledgeable people, who really care about you have been trying to tell you for years what fat is all about, but have you listened?
Noooooo. That's okay. I've got a few greasy skeletons in my closet, too. Everybody does. That's why I'm not even going to slam you about that three-year
affair you had with the whipped-cream can, either.

I'm not here to guilt-gorge you about your weight. In fact, I think women
are fabulous in all shapes and sizes because beauty isn't just a state in the
world of Barbie. If she were a real person, her measurements wouldn't be
39-18-33. (We all know we come in different shapes and sizes.) Trying to look
like Barbie won't help you achieve beauty—it'll just make you nip, tuck, and
run amuck. Just like Barbie, 5'10", 117-pound fashion models are icons of
unreasonable commercialism that can just promote insanity. Models are skin-
nier than 98 percent of all the women in America: hips like boys and Barbie-
doll breasts. Have you ever wondered why those models aren't smiling on

1

the runway? They're hungry, that's why. So it is best to stop starving in an attempt to look like *that*.

Thin has never been *in*—somebody in the 1970s coined that phrase because it rhymed. The only thing I personally want thin is my stack of unpaid bills. Believe me, only a dog wants a bone, and he'll bury it and forget where he put it. Think *lean*, not thin. There's an emaciated world of difference between the two. People should be able to give you a hug without getting splinters.

The average American woman is a sexy, sumptuous 5'4", 143-pound groove-thing with a 39-inch built-in seat cushion. She's got nerve in her curves and would never consider using a Cheerio for a lifesaver. She's also got what the average American man is dying to get his hands on. That's real.

Now, take a deep breath, count to ten, and let it out. It's time for a reality check. I'm talking about total verisimilitude, an honest, no-holds-barred, all-up-in-your-face look at who you are. Ready? Get up and go to your bathroom. Take this book with you. I don't want you to be alone.

Close the door and stand in front of the mirror. Now, take off all your clothes. That's right, *all of them*. Quickly, quickly, before you throw the book away. Makeup, too. Don't worry; there aren't any hidden cameras, so stop looking. Yes, it's okay if you lock the door even though we're the only two here.

Okay, open your eyes and really take a look at yourself from head to toe, right to left, front to back. Take it all in. Do you like what you see?

Talk-show moment: You *can* change yourself anytime you're ready. There is a *you* inside the person you are looking at who is exactly the person you want to be, and she loves you for who you are, right now. She is what I call your Sister-Self—that woman within who is every ambition, dream, goal, idea, and vision you ever had about yourself. You have to get to know her, and the only way to do that is to be honest about who you are. When this happens, the *outside* you and the *inside* you meet. And then—WOW. Every right-out-of-the-shower, full-body mirror-gazing experience you will ever have again will be heavenly.

Now get dressed.

It's a fact: Women spend more time, energy, and emotion building the facade of who they want the world to see rather than discovering and mining the truth of who they really are. Many women live their entire lives in a state of camouflage. They have surgery and cosmetics that reface them, undergarments that reshape them, and fashion tricks that recreate them.

It's time to get real about your body, your weight, your dress size—you. Just because it says *petite* doesn't mean you are. It just means you're shorter than 5'3". You know that, and you also know that today's size 8 is yesterday's size 12. Yeah, but you don't mind the garment industry lying to you about wearing the same dress size, even though you're twenty pounds heavier than you were twenty years ago.

Women get down on men about lying to them, but women lie to themselves every day. Stop asking your guy, *Do these pants make my butt look big?* Excess fat makes your butt look too big. You know that, and no, those pants do not make you look fat. That stuff bulging and dimpling under your pants does.

There are no calories in air. You are not breathing them in. It's one of two things: You're overeating them or you're not eating enough. There are three primary reasons for loading up on fat stores:

1. Excessive calorie intake

2. The wrong percentage of calories from the wrong food categories

3. You're starving, dieting, call it what you want, and you're not eating enough (I see this in 90 percent of the women and teens I counsel)

Let's figure it out together and stop blaming your thyroid. In all my years as a nutritionist, I rarely see an underactive thyroid cause a weight gain of more than 10–20 pounds. And a good percentage of this weight is water and bloat that can be exorcised by sweating daily, drinking *enough* water, and consuming enough fuel daily to support your base caloric needs. So, that 40, 50, 80 pounds you've been using to make your thyroid the scapegoat, well, just call me the whistle blower who is keeping it real.

One more thing. Your thyroid doesn't have a brain. It doesn't make choices. It has no control over you not providing your body with enough fuel daily, or your choosing to eat a whole box of frozen cream puffs while you watch *Desperate Housewives* in your sweatpants. Besides, if you embrace the concept of lights out by 10 P.M., sleep at least eight hours every night, drink ample water, eat two to four cups of vegetables and some fruit every day (strawberry cheesecake doesn't count), and stop mainlining all that coffee and diet soda into your bloodstream, your thyroid will be just fine. A trot around the block a couple of times a week will help activate your thyroid and metabolism as well. Think: woefully poor choices, not underactive gland.

Yes, I know there are numerous studies showing that weight gain and obesity can be genetically influenced. I've read them. I concede the connection, but stop blaming the bagel-and-fries eating on your parents. They may have been in charge of feeding you once, but they're not force-feeding you now.

The penalty for eating too many *side orders* of fries could be a trip to the cardiac intensive care unit down the road. And that kind of a *side* doesn't come with ketchup.

Also, you cannot look at food and get fat. That's a big ol' lie. You can no more look at food and get fat than you can look at a diamond ring and get engaged. Try that the next time you go to Tiffany & Co. Stand at the counter and eyeball that four-carat emerald cut in the platinum setting and see if Mr. Right shows up. Don't think so.

Now try a little word association. *Honesty* and *healthy* both start with the letter *h*. *Denial*, and *damn, look how tight my pants are* both start with the letter *d*. You are the only one who pays the pound penalty for lying to yourself, no one else. The flip side: You are also the only one who gets the beauty bonus and the wellness windfall from being truthful about where you're at with your body fat.

There are two kinds of people in the world: Those who think they can, and those who think they can't—and they're both right. They key word here is *think*. Translation: Ultimately, the battle of your bulge must be won before you pick up your fork. Hand-to-mouth is a brain-guided activity. Change how you think, expand your awareness, and you'll alter—for the better—how you eat, what you eat, how often you eat, and why you eat. You might even be compelled to shake your bootie with exercise.

Everyone knows that controlling fat and creating a lean body isn't just about food and eating, right? I know it's not easy dining at the reality table. A serving of truth can be tough to chew and even tougher to swallow. But you're not reading this book to find a pound-cake recipe, so I'm not going to marshmallow you about what's happening with your hips or thighs. Understand that the first step to new thinking is being honest with yourself, always.

That's why I want you to spend at least five minutes at the start of each day totally naked in front of a mirror, and really look at yourself. You'll never have a more honest moment.

And while you're there, ask yourself this question: What am I going to do today to become who I want to be?

If you do this, you will begin to see your Sister-Self looking back at you. Talk to her. Get to know her. Then treat her to some love and a good facial or massage versus a pint of Chunky Monkey. Seventy-five percent of the women I counsel lack self-care. You may love ice cream, but you won't get hugs from that container. You will get some concentrated calories that will concentrate on making love to your fat cells while clogging up an artery or two or three. It may take a year or ten, but eventually your most frequent late-night conversations will be with your physician. If you want to stroll down the red carpet of lean health and beauty, then stop ignoring your Sister-Self.

There's fortified nutrition in truth. It's time to give your soul a dose. If you want your true *you* to emerge in all of her heart-healthy, here-I-am glory, then reach out to your Sister-Self. She's got nothing but love for you, and unlike some of your other friends, she will never lie to you.

You're More Than a Number

*D*id you know that Christopher Columbus didn't discover America? I kid you not. He never set foot in Washington, D.C. He believed the world was round (give him credit) and set out to prove it by sailing west to get to India, which everyone knew was east of Spain. Then he got lost and, as is all-too-typically male, wouldn't stop to ask for directions and wound up drifting down the coast of Africa and across the ocean until he landed on some islands in the Caribbean Sea. Thinking he had in fact proven his point by landing in India, *his* new world came to be known as the West Indies. Now you're asking yourself, what can this possibly have to do with me getting real about my weight? A ton.

The world doesn't run on truth. It runs on perceptions, which are view-points processed by the filters of personal experience and molded by the motivations of other people. In politics, it's called spin, as in, *Let me spin your head this way and show you this. It's important for you to believe this.* People don't even look for truth in the courtroom. The justice system is based on reasonable doubt, and that's not the same thing as absolute truth. Reasonable doubt means, *What can I convince you of?*

Women have developed a warped perception about weight scales. With great conviction, they have allowed themselves to be convinced that when they step on them, scales have an almighty ability to determine whether or not they're living in heaven or hell. The numbers registered by these density demigods are perceived as absolute indicators of how healthy and how beautiful women are. Wrong. If you are ever to be free from worrying about your weight, you must come to terms with this truth about numbers:

Scales only tell you how much you weigh.

A scale cannot differentiate between pounds of bloat, bone, clothing, fat, feces, muscle, or water. Scales don't tell you how many pounds of self-esteem you have, or the kilogram weight of your many talents. They don't tell you if you're a good mother or wife; if you have breast implants, premenstrual bloat, or are pregnant. They don't measure your cholesterol or your personal genius, and they sure don't measure your loveliness and spirit. Besides, you were a *10* when you were born. All babies are adorable. You just need to hook onto that *I'm an adorable 10* mindset once again. I personally abdicated from weighing myself weekly when I stopped modeling years ago. Now I weigh myself twice a year max—in the summer and winter. Talk about liberating!

Did you know that 15 percent of your body's weight is skin? Add another 15 percent for your bones, which sort of kills the I-have-big-bones idea. Fifty to 60 percent of your weight is fluid: blood, water, lymph, green tea, champagne. Your liver weighs three pounds. You have 600 muscles and more than 60,000 miles of blood vessels. The scale can't even *begin* to decipher what all of that weighs.

The point is that weight can be anything. Gas is weight. You can wake up in the morning after eating a bowl of refried beans the previous night and feel five pounds heavier. Get a divorce and you can drop 20 pounds of *Whew, glad that's over,* just like that. Girlfriend, you can lose weight if you get a short enough haircut.

It is important that you realize you are far more than a number on a scale, because that number doesn't fully reflect your state of health or define your value as a human being. Case in point: The total market value of all the physical ingredients that make up the average person is $4.50. That's what the scale measures. Now, you have to believe that your value as an individual is more than $4.50, so:

Stop measuring your self-worth on the scale.

BODY FAT MEASUREMENTS

The issue isn't how much your *body* weighs. The issue is how much your *fat* weighs. Fat is why people avoid full-length mirrors. Fat is why you only have sex when the lights are out. Fat is what's putting pressure on your heart, pestering your liver, and pounding your knees and back into submission.

Did you know that one pound of fat can take up five times as much space as one pound of muscle? Muscle is dense and compact. It's like comparing corn puffs to gold nuggets. You need a shoulder bag to carry a pound of corn puffs, but a pound of gold can fit in the palm of your hand. This is why you could be the same height and weight as another woman who has more body fat than you and still wear a smaller dress size than she does. Less body fat means you take up less space in your clothes. The scale can't determine your dress size, either.

The average American woman, that 5'4", 143-pound sweet thing with a 39-inch tush, generally carries 28 to 30 percent of her body weight as fat. More ideal (we're talking about reducing health risk and improving looks) would be 23 to 25 percent fat. If more than one-fourth of your weight, 35 to 40 percent, can be measured as fat, you bear the burden of having legitimately excess body fat. This means the average American woman needs to ask herself how much verve in her curves she really needs. Twenty-nine percent and above moves you toward mildly high body fat while the ideal is 18 to 25 percent. For most women, obesity starts at approximately 32 percent.

To calculate your pounds of fat, you will need to plug your body-fat percentage into the following equation:

$$\text{Weight} \times \text{body-fat percent} = \text{pounds (lbs) of fat}$$
$$\text{Example: } 143 \times 28 \text{ percent} = 40.0 \text{ lbs of fat}$$

Despite the alarming reality it might verify, it's important to have your percentage of body fat checked. I know what you are saying: *I don't need to know that much about myself.* Oh, but you do because too much fat can lead to:

- Adult-onset diabetes
- Alzheimer's disease
- Arthritis
- Blood clots

- Clogged arteries
- Congestive heart failure
- Dermatitis
- Gallstones
- Gout
- Heart attacks
- Hypertension
- Infertility

- Insulin resistance
- Kidney stones
- Ovarian cysts
- Sleep apnea
- Stroke
- A variety of cancers: breast, colon, endometrial, esophageal, kidney, and rectal

These health problems are a lot worse than dimples, stretch marks and cellulite. Bottom dimples and rolls of back fat may be unsightly, but it isn't fat's appearance that will kill you, so check your fat percentage.

You can have your body fat measured by a physician, healthcare practitioner, or fitness professional. The most common test procedures are skin-fold caliper testing, bioelectrical impedance, and hydrostatic weighing. Here's a breakdown on each method and how they do what they do.

Skin-Fold Calipers

This is a pinch-an-inch test and the most widely used method (I use it on my clients). A skin-fold caliper (large, lobster-claw-looking tweezers) is used to pinch (not painfully) different areas of the body to measure fat folds against muscle mass. The sites typically measured are: triceps (the too floppy skin on the back of the arm), subscapular (the backup bust line under the shoulder blade), suprailiac (the not-so-Goodyear spare tire), abdomen (the midriff mush), and sometimes the thigh (feel the thunder). Your fat-fold measurements (recorded in centimeters) are applied to a mathematical formula, which yields the magic number—your body-fat percentage.

The upside is that the test is cheap ($10–$20), can be done quickly (two to five minutes), and has a relatively low margin of error if done correctly (± 3 percent). The downside is that it has the potential for faulty measurements, increasing the margin of error (by as much as 8 percent), if done by an inexperienced tester. If you choose this method, make sure the tester has at least 100 examinations under her or his belt. There are some other things to consider as well.

- Don't exercise directly before the test. If you think this will give you a better percentage result, you're wrong. When you exercise, blood flushes into your skin, making it temporarily thicker. You don't want thicker skin right before you do a *skin*-fold test.

- Don't oil or lotion up before testing. This makes it hard for the tester to get a good pinch grip, and you'll end up with a higher percentage than you expected. This is not the time to be thinking about moisturizing.

- Keep in mind that you will have to get partially undressed to allow access to the measuring sites and the tester will be pinching fat on various parts of your body. Given that the tester could be a woman or a man, you should think about your comfort level with this beforehand. If you prefer a woman, seek her out.

- Note that the mathematical formula used to calculate your measurements is based on the assumption that 50 percent of your body fat is subcutaneous—stored under the skin. This isn't true for everyone, however. Some people have very little fat stored under their skin, but have more stored in and around the muscles and internal organs (tan-colored visceral fat). If you have more tan fat you tend to have a harder time than most losing weight, therefore, you might want to consider another method. Also, the test isn't very useful for people who are very obese because the caliper claws only open so wide.

If you choose the skin-fold method, use the same test person for all follow-ups to insure consistency.

Bioelectrical Impedance

Relax, it's not shock therapy. You don't feel a thing. Some people fall asleep during it. You can even do it if you're pregnant, but why would you? If you're pregnant or nursing, a body-fat test, just like a diet, shouldn't even register on your radar screen of concern. Get the nursery ready. Enjoy those months of sweet reprieve.

Bioelectrical impedance is based on the principle that water is a good conductor of electricity. You know this, which is why you don't blow-dry your hair while you're rinsing off in the shower.

A muscle cell is about 75 percent water. By comparison, a fat cell is 10 to 13 percent water. So, if you send a *harmless* electrical current through your body and measure how fast it travels, you can get an estimate of how much fat you have. Since fat has less water, it impedes—slows down—the current.

This test costs a bit more than the skin-fold test ($30–$40), takes about twice as long to do (four to ten minutes) and has a comparable margin of error (±3 percent). You don't have to worry about the tester's experience level influencing the outcome, as the tester is a machine. However, there are some guidelines to follow to reduce error.

- Don't eat or drink for at least four hours before the test. This could influence how much water (hence fat) appears to be in your body.

- Don't exercise at least twelve hours before testing—same reason.

- Don't consume alcohol for at least forty-eight hours before testing—again, same reason.

- Urinate at least thirty minutes before your test.

- Don't consume diuretics for at least seven days before testing—it's a water thing.

Sometimes the test is done standing barefoot on metal plates while the current is sent up one leg and down the other. Other times it's done while reclining and the current is passed through electrodes attached to a hand and a foot. Either way, you are going to have to take your socks off. Also, this method tends to overestimate body fat for lean people and underestimate it for obese people, so its reliability is a bit fickle and open to question.

Some bioelectrical impedance scales are available for home use. If you choose to get one, stick to the guidelines mentioned to insure better self-testing. Otherwise, you'll find yourself in a high-body-fat-error rage, throwing the machine to the floor and wasting your money.

Hydrostatic Weighing

This is considered the gold standard for measuring body fat. The test is based upon the Archimedean principle, named for Archimedes, the famous guy of Greek origin, even though he was born in Sicily. Anyway, several millennia ago, Archimedes figured out that if you plunge an object into water, it will become lighter by an amount equal to the weight of water it displaces. He also came up with a formula to calculate the weight of the displaced water, and this is used in hydrostatic weighing. By the way, Archimedes figured this out when he stepped into a bathtub (which is where I do a lot of my figuring out). He was so excited about his buoyant discovery that he went running into the street yelling, "Eureka!" Yep, he was the father of that too.

In case you haven't figured it out it yet, you will have to get wet to do this test because *you* will be the object going into the water (no, not nude). Your lean mass (bones, muscles, internal organs, etc.) is far denser than water and fat. If you have more lean mass than fat mass, you will weigh more when you get into the tub. That's a good thing. Fat floats, so if you have more fat mass, you will weigh less in the water. That's a not-so-good thing. When it comes to hydrostatic weighing, more means less, and less means more.

This is the most expensive of the tests mentioned (it can be as much as $75, or can be found as low as $20 in some health clubs). It takes longer to administer (fifteen to twenty minutes) but has the lowest margin of error ($\pm$ 1.5 percent). As with the other methods described, there are some guidelines and influencing factors to consider before taking the plunge.

- If you can't handle being underwater for a few seconds, or you don't want to get your hair wet, don't do it.

- The degree of accuracy depends on how well you can blow all the air out of your lungs (through a tube) while underwater. You see, air makes the body float, and you want to reduce any floatation caused by air in order to measure the amount of flotation from fat.

This test requires a lot of space and equipment so it's not as readily available as the others. You will have to do some looking around to find a hydrostatic weighing set-up. Your best chances are at a top-end fitness facility, a university (especially if it's big on sports), or a really good hospital. Also, have it done only by individuals who are well trained in administering the test and doing the calculations.

An autopsy is absolutely the most accurate way to measure body fat. I'm sure you're not opting for this procedure just yet, however. So don't expedite your untimely demise in a portly manner. Have your body fat measured to help place you on the path of a longer, leaner, healthier life.

BODY MASS INDEX (BMI)

Another popular number to get tagged with is your body mass index (BMI). This calculation is based on weight-to-height ratios. You can figure out your BMI with this simple formula:

$$(\text{weight} \div \text{height}^2) \times 703 = \text{BMI}$$

Using this formula for the average American woman, we get:

$$(143 \text{ pounds} \div 64^2 \text{ inches}) \times 703 = 24.5$$

What does this mean? Well, based on BMI indexes from the World Health Organization (WHO) and the Centers for Disease Control (CDC), having a BMI under 18 is considered being underweight, a BMI from 18.5 to 24.9 is considered healthy, and 25 to 29.9 is marginally overweight to overweight, while anything over 30 is obese.

Here's the interesting thing. According to this index, the weight of the average American woman is within the healthy range, even though her body fat percentage indicates she is fat. As I said before, forget about the Barbie-supermodel myth. Weight alone will not tell you the whole story. You can be a vivacious 5'4", 143-pound, 16 percent-body-fat poster child for sexy health, slinking around town in a size 6. You can also be a 5'4", 143-pound, 35-percent body-fat medical-jeopardy queen, thumbing through the full-size racks looking for coverage. Same height, same weight, but different dress sizes. What your weight is made up of is more important than its scale value. Lean, not thin or skinny, is the goal.

Although your BMI can be a good indicator of health risks relative to weight and height ratios, it still doesn't tell you what your risks are relative to how much fat you have. That's more important. Some very lean, muscular people have very high BMIs, but they have nowhere near the health risks of people with higher body-fat percentages. Also, BMI is a less accurate indicator of health risk when associated with weight for people under 5 feet, or for older people, who tend to lose bone and muscle mass as they age.

WAIST-TO-HIP RATIO (WHR)

There is yet another way to measure yourself, and many health experts feel it is better than the BMI. But before I tell you what it is, have you ever heard of an omentum? No, it has nothing to do with the potential or influence of force. That's momentum. Everybody has an omentum. It's a squishy, gushy, cushy organ made up of arteries, veins, connective tissue, lymphatics, and fat pads, and it encases your bowel, as well as everything from the stomach down to the rectum. So, think of your omentum as a brisket basket (the fatty layer in a brisket) for your gut. Bear with me now.

There was a huge study (with more than 10,000 people) done between 1988 and 1994 by the National Center for Health Statistics. It was called NHANES III, which stands for National Health and Nutrition Examination Survey. One of the most profound revelations to come out of this very important study has to do with comparing apples and pears.

Some women have a tendency to store fat around their hips. They're pear shaped. Other women store more fat around their middle, which makes them apple shaped—oh me, oh my, omentum. Now the NHANES III study showed that apples are at greater risk for diabetes and cardiovascular disease than pears. Why? I'll tell you.

Even though visceral fat (the tan fat surrounding the internal organs) that contributes to an apple-shaped body only accounts for 20 percent or less of your total body fat, it's metabolically more active. Its proximity to your organs means it has more blood-vessel innervation, which means more fat ends up in your bloodstream. The fat on your hips is less accessible and therefore more likely to stay out of your bloodstream until you actually need it. So, it's better to be a pear than an apple. All big-butt girls (me included) stand and take a bow.

Furthermore, in the study the waist measurements proved to be far superior predictors of health risk when compared to the BMI. Consequently the National Institutes of Health (NIH), CDC, and *American Journal of Clinical Nutrition* all recommend keeping your waist under 35 inches for women, 40 inches for men. The CDC even came up with an assessment indicator to help monitor waist circumference relative to health risk. It's called the waist-to-hip ratio (WHR).

To figure your WHR, grab a tape measure and divide your waist measurement by your hip measurement. This is much easier than being pinched or dunked. To properly measure your waist, wrap the tape measure around the *biggest* part of your midsection. To properly measure your hips, wrap the tape measure around the *biggest* part of your tush. Take your measurements and divide. As long your WHR is less than .80, you're okay. Anything higher and you're asking for it. The average American woman has a 32–34-inch waist, giving her a WHR of .82 to .87.

Researchers at the British Columbia Cancer Agency, the University of British Columbia, and the University of Washington (all contributors to NHANES III) found that for every tenth of a point increase in WHR, that's .10 mind you, postmenopausal women had a 40-percent greater risk of mortality. In other words, if a woman goes from .80 to .90, that's a 40-percent risk increase; and going from .80 to 1 is an 80-percent risk increase. The *American Heart Journal* in January 2005 backed this up by reporting that for every increase of .01 above a WHR of .83, women show a 4-percent increase for cardiovascular death, a 4-percent increase for myocardial infarction (heart attack), and a 5-percent increase for heart failure.

Here's what I advise: Never let your waist measure more than your inseam. Follow this guide and your waist will always be 60 to 80 percent smaller than your hips, which will keep you in a WHR range of .60 to .80. You'll get the health benefit of keeping your waist size down and an aesthetic appearance that will be more appreciated. With a waist circumference equal to, or less than, the length of your inseam, you could end up with a *drop 10*. In fashion parlance this means having a waist that measures 10 inches less than your bust. No doubt a waist 10 inches smaller than your bust will also be close to 10 inches smaller than your hips. For example, a 36-26-36 figure will yield a WHR of .72. In the parlance of sexy, that's a show-stopper. More curves, better health—a win-win situation.

New thinking for a new you: Ditch the scale. Your body-fat percentage (< 25 percent), body mass index (< 25), and waist-to-hip ratio (< .80) actually mean something. Use them instead.

Diets, and Lies, and Thighs, Oh My!

*W*ant to get rich quick? Come up with some kind of fad diet or magic weight-loss pill because Americans spend $40 billion a year dieting. That's billions with a *b*! Why so much money? Because . . . diets don't work.

Now, you all know this, but you keep trying new ones anyway, and every time you buy the quick-weight-loss books, pills, products, and programs, the diet industry expands and hauls in the bucks. Ca-ching—$$$. And what happens to you? You also expand by packing on more fat. One definition of insanity is doing the same thing over and over again and expecting a different result each time. Does this make any sense? Of course not. So why keep trying new improved diets and insane fat-burning cures?

Almost half the women in this country are chronic dieters (CDs), women who are always trying to lose the same ten pounds, which turn into twenty and then thirty because they just keep getting bigger after each ride on the diet-go-round. OK, think about this. The two most enjoyed activities in life are sex and eating. Which ranks first for most women? Hint: You can't get pregnant from doing it.

I'm all about spending some prime time on cloud nine with someone hunky and divine, but for most, good food is number one. The upside is being able to chow down virtually anytime without requiring a partner's participation to achieve satisfaction. On the other hand, the downside of these self-induced culinary orgasms is being able to chow down virtually anytime to achieve them. See the problem? How can you restrict what is arguably the most enjoyed activity in the realm of human experience? Why should you when it gives you such delicious pleasure? Talk about an uphill battle.

It's easy to get caught up in that whole *Yes! Yes! Oh, my God! Oh, my God! I'm eeeaaaating!* thing. Women often eat for reasons that have nothing to do with hunger. Bored? Eat. Happy? Eat. Just got fired? Meet me for lunch. Just got hired? Dinner, my treat. Women overeat because something is lacking. They undereat because they're too busy. They diet as a lifestyle, embracing starvation and a no-fat life as a good hug. Pass your real estate test? How about a hot fudge sundae? Flunked the Bar exam? Starve all day, and then . . . How about a box of cookies? Or a bubbly Diet Coke accompanied by a salty plate of chips or fries?

Pay attention because it's really important to get this. Food is not a pill to rid yourself of emotional anxieties; it's not an ointment to heal your relationship wounds; and it's definitely not Matthew McConaughey and Taye Diggs rolled up into one, gazing into your eyes . . . you get the point.

Eat for one reason and one reason only: because you're hungry. If you're hungry all the time, then either you have a metabolic condition that needs further diagnosis or you have other appetites that aren't getting fed, and that's a different book, so let's move on.

This may surprise you. Dieting as you have come to think of it is one of the best ways to get fat. No, really. Why? Let me give you the skinny laced with a little anthropology lesson.

Hundreds of thousands of years ago, when women were still running from saber-toothed tigers and ape-like men without deodorant (or was that last week?), long before Peapod, an online grocery delivery service, the drive-through window, and caramel-mocha lattes, their bodies had to figure out ways to keep them alive. One way was the development of two separate fuel systems.

Our metabolism operates a bit like today's hybrid cars, but instead of using gas and electricity, it uses carbohydrates and fat. Carbohydrates are just a bunch of sugars strung together. Relative to fat, carbohydrates are fairly easy to break down and digest, which is why they are readily available as energy floating around in the veins and arteries. Hence, the term blood sugar (glucose, to be exact). Are you still with me? Good.

Now, since this carbohydrate fuel is so easy to access, it gets used for all of your short-term activities—blow-drying your hair, putting on makeup, running the kids around; all these activities are fueled readily by carbohydrates, the short-term fuel for your body. If too many excess carbohydrates are consumed, they store as reserve fuel for up to twelve hours after overconsumption. Then, they store as fat.

Fat is a more concentrated fuel, which is why it yields nine calories per gram versus the four calories that come from a gram of carbohydrates. Fat is also a slower burning fuel. Fats vary, so depending on the type of fat, it takes a bit more effort for your metabolism to break fat down, digest it, and make it available for use, which is why, if it is a *good* fat, it can help to burn stored *bad* fats. Think of those hunks of fat hanging around your waistline as reserve saturated-fat fuel tanks. Oh, so now you finally want to jump on the alternative fuel bandwagon.

Since fat is stored fuel, it isn't as accessible in the bloodstream as carbohydrates. You have to burn off the carbohydrates before you can tap the fat stores (more about this later). So fat only gets used during long-term activities—all-day Saturday laundry and housecleaning; an afternoon reorganizing your closets and throwing nothing away; two hours of over-the-top, break-the-box springs, Samantha-Jones sex; all these are fueled by fat, the long-term fuel for your body. Where am I going with this?

Again, let's go back to pre-online shopping days, before people began cultivating crops, raising hormone-laden, stressed-out livestock, and picking out men on e-Harmony. Back then, when people were nomads, they were hunter-gatherers living off the land, foraging here, scavenging there, hunting to and fro, and sometimes going for hours, even days, without eating. Unfortunately, far too many women I encounter still do this. During food shortages, bodies learned to *sloooow* down, conserve energy, and rely on reserved fuel—fat—to get through these periods of calorie deprivation.

Did you see the movie *March of the Penguins*? I love any movie with Morgan Freeman's voice in it. Anyway, remember how the daddy penguins had to stand around caring for their eggs for three months without eating? Amazing.

They had to rely on their fat reserves to get them through that tough time. Different animal. Same thing.

For the hunter-gatherers, when food became available again and the calorie deprivation cycle was over (yippee), people's bodies learned to convert most initial calorie intake into fat to replenish depleted energy reserves for the next time of going without. That's why penguins get fat again and bears pig-out before hibernating. It's similar to stocking up with a twelve-pack of Pepsi or a triple-pack of Pringles. And where do reserves get put? You got it— on the backs of arms, on breasts, around the middle, and in the saddlebags. These are the body's food pantries.

While talking about stocking up, let me share these facts with you: One pound of fat equals 454 grams, so every pound of fat your body stores represents 4,086 calories of unused energy (454 grams/lbs $\times$ 9 calories/gram).

Your body stores your fat in your fat cells. You are born with 80 to 100 billion of them. Think of yourself as a walk-in closet with 80 to 100 billion built-in storage cubicles, all holding blubber blobs instead of shoes. Here's the real kicker. Women can increase the number of their fat cells many more times than men, as toddlers, as teens in puberty, and during pregnancy when many fat cells fill up and reach maximum capacity, split, divide into new ones, and start filling up again. Of all the nerve. So, while you're playing the poker game no limit Texas hold 'em with your waistline, your fat-cell chip count keeps getting bigger and bigger. This is not a good thing. You can't cash in your fat cells for a new Lexus. Depending on how many pregnancies you've had during your lifetime, you can double, even quadruple your fat-cell numbers. That can gear you toward full-tilt obesity.

Back to the facts. The stocking-of-energy-reserves survival mechanism is called the feast-or-famine response, or the thrifty gene, due to its ability to store calories when food is scarce. Since survival is the strongest motivation around, this is a pretty compelling mechanism. It's one of the reasons your body craves fatty foods when you start dieting. You see, your fat cells aren't just sitting around on their big bubble butts taking up space. They're a lot like politicians, always hitting you up for the next contribution, and the more fat cells you reproduce and fill, the greedier they get.

These greedy little bad boys don't really give a hoot about your clogged arteries, or your diabetes, or what you look like in lingerie. To them, it's all about feeding the fat stores—the more, the better. So, when you switch allegiance to the Non-Eating party, they switch to their get-out-the-vote telemarketing strategy. They employ an army of loyal campaign workers—proteins, hormones and neurotransmitters—all manning the fat phones twenty-four hours a day with one goal: to get you to eat . . . more and soon!

These lard-talking lackeys will dial you up at all hours of the day and night, trying to woo your vote with a junket to Dunkin' Donuts. And they have the nerve to get indignant on your appetite voicemail if you ignore them: *Hey, we worked our plump rumps off to get you one more chin. You owe us. Make a contribution—say, a whopper order of fries, with lots of ketchup, of course.*

Then you fall off the wagon, blame yourself for having no willpower, and spend the next three months on a chocolate-chip-cookie guilt trip. It's not your fault. You can't override a prehistoric, built-in survival mechanism without a little know-how. Don't worry, that's what I'm here for . . . stay close.

Check this out. It has been scientifically determined that the feast-or-famine response will engage the moment that your daily caloric intake drops *below 1,200 calories.* That's the bare minimum for most women. Whether you wear a size 4 or a size 14, the fat-storage button gets cranked on at 1,199. But did you know that most lose-ten-pounds-in-ten-days or raw-food diets will take you down to 900, 700, even 500 calories a day, for as long as two to four weeks? I don't know about you, but I'm built like a Bentley, not a Volkswagon. I need a full tank of gas. Six hundred calories won't propel anyone out of the garage and up the ramp.

This is just one of the reasons you can drink diet sodas all day long and still be fat. If you don't eat enough calories, your metabolism will *slooooow* down and you'll go back to being a Neanderthal woman. All that diet, fat-free fluff you're psyching yourself out with is just artificially filling you up and setting you up for a buns' worth of trouble. Oh, by the way, you're wearing a double-D denial mindset if you really think that stuff offsets the other calorific junk you're eating. That whole Big Mac/Diet Coke thing makes about as much sense as smashing your thumb in a car door in order to offset a migraine.

Hopefully, this is all beginning to make sense. It's important to remember

that every time you go on a cabbage soup, cayenne pepper, honey, and grape-
fruit only, low-fat, no-fat, or totally-raw-food-only diet, inducing a hunger
strike, you trigger the body's fat-storage response. Your metabolism then
slooooows down—again—to get you through this self-induced famine. Your
body morphs into an angry wife at 3 A.M., waiting for the wayward food to
show up. You'll lose weight all right, most of it being lean tissue and water.
Then, the moment you stop dieting and start eating again, with intuitive
sense your body quickly restores the lean tissue and water weight because you
need it. That's why it's called *essential* weight. Then the cave-woman thing
kicks in. Your fat-storing mechanism slams into overdrive and you start
stockpiling fat all over again.

You are an evolved human being with credit cards, a Blackberry, and a
401K. You watch Oprah. You use feng shui just in case it works. You know
what the flashing red light on the dashboard means, and you know this country is ready for a female president with common sense. So lose the simian attitude. *Diets only teach your body to store fat.*

Please hear this. Put down that bagel and listen to me. If you keep dieting,
you're going to earn a Ph.D. in body-fat storage. In the end, your rear end to
be exact, all the weight will come back, plus a fat bonus. Then you're bound
up in the yo-yo diet. Gain, lose, gain, lose, gain, lose.

Don't fear your fat weight. Know it and understand it, because once you
understand it you will know what to do about it. Eventually your body gets
fed up (pun intended) with the stress of all the weight-gain and weight-loss
fluctuations and it then crashes like the stock market in 1929. You're left with
a gluteus maximus depression and, let me tell you . . . there's no government
bailout for getting behind in body-fat build-up. I've checked.

Dieting is a complete waste of time. And no one has the time to waste.
Everyone has too much to do—children to love and nurture, money to make,
vacations to take, the perfect relationship to find, and a clearance sale to hit.
Lose the diets.

Media alert: Diet is a noun, not a verb. It isn't a ride at the amusement
park. It's not something you're supposed to keep going on and getting off.
And it sure isn't some nouveau chic tabloid-magazine, calorie-counting man-
ifesto designed to drive you insane, and alienate you from all your friends and

social functions for weeks on end. Here is the only definition for the word *diet* you will ever need. *Diet is the food and drink you consume to satisfy hunger, quench thirst, and promote optimum health—period.*

This means that a diet is an eating lifestyle. New concept? Not really. The eating lifestyle in Japan is different than it is in Brazil, which is different than it is in Sweden, which is different than it is in Sao Tomé and Principe (check out an atlas). There are many cultures around the world with just as many interpretations on food. Eating lifestyles (diets) vary from region to region in this country. That's what a diet is. How the word ever came to mean beauty by starvation is beyond me.

The issue now is what kind of eating lifestyle you have. If you have a bacon double-cheeseburger, large fries, 48-ounce Diet-Coke eating lifestyle, you'll probably end up fitting into a piano box at your funeral. On the other hand, if you have an eating lifestyle of coldwater fish or tenderloin, accompanied by half a plate of colorful vegetables drizzled with lots of olive oil, a serving of starch the size of a small apple, plus water with a lime, you'll fit nicely into that haute couture self-esteem with the scandalous watch-me-strut hemline. If you are confused, I'll go with you back to page one and your mirror.

Diets promise to help you lose weight and they do. But weight, as I explained earlier, can be anything. What you're interested in losing is *fat*. That's the stuff doing the muffin top over your low-rise jeans. That's the deep-fried high-cholesterol chicken winging it's way through your arteries. Think about it. Diets = weight loss. Have you ever heard of a diet that promised to help you lose fat? No, because you can't lose ten pounds of fat in a week. That would really be a big lie—a big, fat one.

Here's one more thing to think about. You don't need to go on a diet to trigger your feast-or-famine response. Just skip breakfast. Yep, that's right. Your body will respond to a missed meal the same way it reacts to the famine caveman diet. It's calorie deprivation. Get it? Every time you skip a meal or wait too long to eat, your metabolism *sloooows* down and turns on the fat-storage button. I see it coming—mirror avoidance.

So you see, it's not just an issue of staying above 1,200 calories a day. It's also an issue of percentages and the time lapse between feedings. This is why all of those *I am woman* magazines say:

- Don't ever skip breakfast.

- Eat soon after rising.

- Eat smaller meals (five to six) more frequently throughout the day, preferably every two to three hours.

- Stop avoiding healthy-for-you fats.

Remember, you were born with 80 to 100 billion fat cells and that's all you'll ever need in a lifetime. No more diets, no more skipped meals, and no more low-fat or no-fat anything.

Stick to
Your Budget

I once read in a newspaper article that it costs four times more to be a woman than to be a man, which wouldn't be so bad if women made four times the money that men do. Right now, women are still only earning about eighty cents on the male dollar. This is why women are better at budgeting than men. They have to be just to survive the disparity.

Every day when you go to the ATM, you know how much money you can take out. Why? Because you know how much you put in. You know what your available funds are because you keep track of your receipts, read your statements, and balance your accounts, right? You don't overdraw. That's also why you limit your everyday spending. You take out $20 at a time, not $60, because if you take out $60, you'll spend it. That's called fiscal responsibility (you'd need a ballistics expert to find that in Congress).

Now, think of calories as food currency you take from your ATM—your calorie ATM. Every time you eat something, you make a withdrawal to buy its calorie content, so you know how much it's going to cost you. And if you know how much you have to spend for the day, then you know how much to budget for each meal. Make sense?

Now, if your calories per diem is a minimum of 1,200 and you start off with a three-egg, cheddar-cheese omelet, hash browns, and an order of bacon, then you're already close to blowing most of your allotment. You don't want to overdraw on calories. If you do, your metabolism is overfed, in the red, and your backside will be doing the bouncing, not your checks. Conversely, if you only eat a yogurt and cup of coffee for breakfast, you're not putting the bucks into your account for future withdrawals.

It's important to budget your intake. It's important to contribute enough to your calorie account.

Of course, it would be helpful to know how much you actually have to spend every day. This intake amount is known as your basal metabolic rate (BMR). The trendier types prefer the term resting energy expenditure (REE). Either way, think of this as your housekeeping account because it's the amount of calories your body needs to get through the day, even if all you do is sit around the house.

The two most frequently used methods for estimating BMR intake are the Harris-Benedict equation and the Mifflin formula. The Harris-Benedict equation (sounds like a prenuptial calculation) was developed in 1919. It's a bit outdated, which is why it doesn't account for lean body mass. Generically, it's a good start, but if you're a woman with a lot of muscle, this isn't the right method for you. The more comprehensive, and more recently developed, Mifflin formula is favored by healthcare practitioners. Its formula is:

$$\text{BMR} = (10 \times \text{weight in kilograms}) + (6.25 \times \text{height in centimeters}) - (5 \times \text{age in years}) - 161.$$

Stop complaining about the math. It only takes a couple of minutes to do this, and if you're not worth two to three minutes of your own time, then you've just about disowned your Sister-Self. How do you think that makes her feel? Don't use your cell phone calculator. It doesn't factor out enough after the decimal point. Now, divide your weight in pounds by 2.2 to get the kilogram (kg) equivalent.

For the average American woman this means: 143 pounds ÷ 2.2 pounds/ kg = 65 kg.

Next, multiply your height in inches by 2.54 to get the centimeter (cm) equivalent: 64 inches × 2.54 cm/inch = 162.6 cm.

Then multiply your age in years by 5. Since the last Census Bureau Report (2000) lists the median age of American women at 36.6 years, let's use 37 as her age: 37 × 5 = 185.

So the final calculation is: $(10 \times 65 \text{ kg}) + (6.25 \times 162.6\text{cm}) - (5 \times 37)$ $- 161 = \text{BMR}$. In numbers, this is: $650 + 1{,}016.25 - 185 - 161 = 1{,}320.25$.

You're not done yet. Now you have to multiply this number by one of the following activity factors:

- 1.2 = sedentary (couch potato)
- 1.375 = lightly active (out and about one to three days a week)
- 1.55 = moderately active (moderate exercise three to five days a week)
- 1.75 = very active (strenuous exercise/physical labor six to seven days a week)
- 1.9 = extra active (tough training/very demanding labor six to seven days a week)

The average American woman is lightly active, so $1{,}320.25 \times 1.375 = 1{,}815.3$ calories a day.

Believe it or not, that's a very generous daily caloric allowance. You could do some fast-paced good housekeeping on this amount. Now you're going to feel like I've been holding out on you, but I had to check your level of commitment to this first, so forgive me. If you want a simple, less involved, super-quick way to find out your daily caloric needs, measure it this way.

To *maintain* your current weight:

Multiply your current weight _____ × 12 hours of active living = _____

To *lose* 1 pound of fat per week:

Multiply your current weight _____ × 12 hours of active living = _____
− 500 calories (*minimum* or *bare bones* number of calories you need per day)

To determine the number of calories you need a day to maintain your current weight, multiply your weight by your hours of active living per day: 12, or 14, or 16 (this is *without* exercise considerations), whichever reflects the number of hours of movement performed in your day.

To determine the number of calories you need a day to lose 1 pound of fat or weight per week, follow this same formula, then subtract 500 calories.

This short formula will help you determine your daily caloric needs based on your current weight. The 12 represents the twelve hours of active living most people engage in while they're awake. For example, if you are the average American woman weighing 143 pounds, you will need 1,716 calories per day to sustain your weight if you put 12 hours into a day. That's actually 109.3 calories less than the Mifflin calculation, or about a 6-percent difference. These 100 or so calories are easy to shave off your diet. The average hamburger bun is 120 calories. Consume half the bun and drop sixty useless, high-sugar, empty calories.

Now that you know how to figure out your daily caloric allowance based on your current body weight in pounds (lbs), you can figure it out for your ideal body weight (IBW). If you know this, then you will know how to reallocate your calorie budget for fat reduction. Use the following formulas to help you out:

Ideal body weight (IBW) = 100 lbs + (5 × inches above 5 feet)

The average American woman of 5'4" has an IBW of 100 lbs + (5 × 4 inches) = 120 lbs.

Adjusted weight = (actual weight − IBW) × .25 + IBW

Using the second formula to determine the average woman's adjusted weight you get (143 lbs − 120 lbs) × .25 + 120 lbs = 125.75 lbs.

Now, rounding off to 126 pounds and allowing (10 pounds for different size body frames (small, medium, and large), a woman will have an ideal adjusted body weight range of 116–136 pounds. Just using the simple formula of weight multiplied by 12 for a twelve-hour day of activity, her daily caloric allowance would be:

- Small frame: 116 × 12 = 1,392 calories
- Medium frame: 126 × 12 = 1,512 calories
- Large frame: 136 × 12 + 1,632 calories

If you allow ±8 pounds for the different size frames women have (small, medium, and large), a 5-foot-4-inch woman will have an ideal/adjusted body weight range of 117.75–133.75 pounds. Just try using the simple formula of your weight multiplied by twelve, or try inserting the correct number of hours expended during your daily life which equals your total daily caloric allowance.

Finally, to determine the amount of calories should be devoted to each food group, follow these formulas:

- Protein calories = Total calorie intake ÷ .30 percent
- Fat and oil calories = Total calories needed × .50 percent
- Low-glycemic, high-fiber carbohydrates = 20 percent

(See page 41, Glycemic Index of Carbohydrates for a list of ideal carbohydrates.)

Knowing these formulations, the average American woman can now alter her daily caloric intake to calculate the optimal number of calories needed to achieve the ideal weight for her height and activity level. Caution: Never drop more than 500 calories from your calculated daily intake. A reduction greater than this can trigger your feast-or-famine response.

Well, all right. Now you know how to determine your daily caloric allowance for both your current weight and your ideal weight.

Problem: Do you have any idea what 1,815.3 calories looks like? How about 1,605 or 1,559.54 or 1,413? You probably have no more a visual concept of any of these calorie amounts than you do of Oprah Winfrey's patronage. How are you supposed to get good value for your calories when you don't really comprehend the amount you have to spend?

Solution: Learn the caloric value of food portions and strategically calculate your intake, every day. Yeah, right. Do this and you'll end up neurotic, uptight, and even more confused. Have you seen the size of some of those calorie-counting books? No wonder the Amazon rainforest is in danger. If you have nothing better to do than to sit around thumbing through 700 pages, trying to memorize the caloric value of every food portion you might ever eat, you need to seriously reevaluate the meaning of life. I do this only when I get paid.

Don't get me wrong. It's ideal to have a nutritional awareness about the calorie cost of what you're depositing into your mouth. I'm all for the calorie-per-servings information listed on food packages and even on the menus of some restaurants. Awareness is the first phase of creating change and gaining control. Determining your daily calorie budget is a good thing, too. You should develop some sense of your calorie-spending goals and limits, because some of you eat like you're living off of trust funds. The rest of you lead your bodies to think you are living in Botswana, starving away day after day.

Still, can you eyeball 6 ounces of salmon? How about 14 grams of lentils? Unless you have so much money you can create your own reality and pay somebody to live in and do the counting for you, then fantasy living isn't for you. I started this whole thing off by encouraging all of you to get real, so it's time to be real about this.

You don't need to know the exact caloric value of a one-pound bag of M&Ms to know that it could bankrupt your daily allowance of calories during one soap opera. That's just common sense. The real solution is to *not* keep counting calories, meticulously measuring food, and studiously studying charts, but to get a grip on serving size instead. It's all about percentage control and where your food choices come from.

Hold on to your thighs. Figure 4.1 at right shows you how the ideal food portions should look on your plate for 1,200 calories.

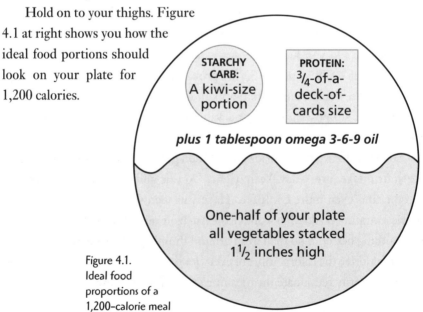

STARCHY CARB: A kiwi-size portion

PROTEIN: 3/4-of-a-deck-of-cards size

plus 1 tablespoon omega 3-6-9 oil

One-half of your plate all vegetables stacked 1 1/2 inches high

Figure 4.1. Ideal food proportions of a 1,200-calorie meal

In the appendices, you'll find tools to help you easily get a handle on your daily calorie intake—one is the Daily Calorie Food Log found in Appendix G. Tracking for three to six weeks works! Use it as a journal to keep track of what, how much, and when you eat. Measurements can be calculated in cups, ounces, or grams. The goal is to *eat*. Eat breakfast, lunch, and dinner, plus three healthy, high-fat snacks throughout the day. Attempt to graze every two to three hours. At breakfast, lunch, and dinner *always* consume a healthy fatty food or oil. Focus on one set of needed changes at a time to create thin thighs. Stick to your plan and ungainly fat will melt by the wayside.

Feed Your Gut
or Feed Your Butt

*A*mericans have a bassackwards sensibility about how much they eat, because they have an economic value associated with the *quantity* of food on the plate, instead of a nutritional health value associated with the *quality* of food on the plate. That's why people think platters and plates the size of toilet-seat covers represent a real meal and a good deal.

Think about this for a moment. Your stomach is the organ that receives food brought in from your mouth. It is about 1.5 times the size of your fist. Go ahead, put your fist right under your diaphragm to create a frame of reference on this. You thought it was bigger, right?

If you think of your stomach as a container, it can comfortably expand to hold 1 to 1.5 liters of fluid. That's roughly a quart to a quart and a half or 34–50 ounces, or for some of you, three to four cans of your favorite diet pick-me-up. Fine bits of trivia I'm giving you, eh?

Remember earlier when I mentioned that the average woman in America had a 39-inch built-in seat cushion? Well, imagine if that bottom were a container. It would hold seven to eight times the amount of your stomach. That's up to 238–350 ounces. Or 7–11 liters. That's nearly 2–3 gallons, and mind you, some bottoms are more than 39 inches around. Here's what I'm getting at.

One of these anatomical containers is going to be the principal or final recipient of what you're shoving down your throat. Stand up right now and make a fist. Plant it next to one of the hemispheres comprising your rear end. Contemplate that size disparity for a moment. It's like comparing the Earth to the moon. Now, perhaps you're ready to hear me on this. When considering food portions and serving sizes, you have a choice to make.

You can feed your gut or you can feed your butt.

This is all you really need to know about serving sizes. It's just that simple. I don't expect you to be able to eyeball 6 ounces of protein, or 22 grams of fat, or 2 cups of carbohydrates. You aren't a forensic scientist. Eating shouldn't be like an episode of *CSI*. However, you can definitely eyeball the difference between a gut-size portion of lean protein and a bottom-size mound of pasta. You don't need measuring cups or food scales for this. All you need is your fist. So, from now on, when you're sizing up what to eat, ask yourself this question: *Am I feeding my gut or am I feeding my butt?*

Good tip: Eat from two smaller plates. Salad size is ideal for your vegetable portion. Cover the entire plate with vegetables, then eat. Your bread plate is the perfect size for your protein and your starchy carbohydrate. Your protein portion should be no larger than a deck of cards, while your starchy carbohydrate portion should be no larger than a kiwi or a very small apple.

The perception of full but smaller plates can help ease the psychological war between sufficient nutrition and overconsumption. You can even do this while dining out. Just ask your server for two salad plates and a takeout container as soon as your meal arrives. Fill up both the smaller plates. That's what you eat from. The rest goes home in the takeout container for a future meal. If you have fairly good self-control, use a large plate, but ask for the take-out container when your meal comes. Half of the larger plate should be the vegetables. Now, that's a nutritional and economical value.

Also, pick up a copy of *The Portion Teller* by Lisa R. Young. This is a great book for teaching you how to eyeball food amounts. Did you know that a 3-ounce chicken breast is visually equal to nearly one deck of playing cards? How about this: three cups of popcorn are equal to six handfuls. Now, that's useful information. This book has all kinds of fun visual references. (*See* Appendix A for additional information on food.)

What's a Girl to Do?

*I*t's so confusing. Everybody is stressing out about making the right decision. Is it high-carbohydrate, low-carbohydrate, or no-carbohydrate—what? Relax. I've got you covered on this, too.

First of all, it's none of these. This whole carbohydrate debate is about as meaningless as an episode of *The Bachelor.* Far more than the amount, the real issue is the *type* of carbohydrate you're putting in your mouth. Here's what I mean.

Carbohydrates have a nutritional personality. There are good simple carbohydrates, such as those found in whole fruits, that are healthier for you and your waist, or there are bad simple carbohydrates, such as the high-fructose corn syrup found in soft drinks and juices and the refined sugars that build thunder thighs—fast.

Simple carbohydrates are comprised of one to three sugars linked together and starchy carbohydrates have three or more sugars linked together. Starch, often contained in seeds, is the form in which plants store energy, and when plants are eaten the starch provides energy. The best starchy carbohydrates are high in fibers that control the release of sugar into your bloodstream.

As their name suggests, simple carbohydrates are easy for your body to quickly digest and break down. Complex carbohydrates, as you might imagine, are a bit more complicated. The body has to spend more time breaking the links holding them together before converting them into blood sugar or glucose. This breakdown occurs in the small intestine and is necessary because only single sugar molecules are small enough to go through the small intestine's openings and enter the bloodstream. This is another reason that all carbohydrates are converted into glucose—it's a single sugar molecule that every cell in the body recognizes as usable fuel. Sugar molecules are also the primary fuel for your brain.

Another reason it takes longer to break down complex carbohydrates is the fiber content. Fiber is also a carbohydrate, but it can't be broken down into sugar. So, your body just gets rid of it in the end, know what I mean? Anyway, think of fiber as an outer coating, like a nutshell. Your digestive enzymes have to crack that shell to get to the sugar inside. This takes time, which *slooooows* down the rate at which sugar enters the bloodstream, and that is the main issue in a nutshell. How much time it takes the body to convert your carbohydrate of choice into sugar is the real question to ask.

If this conversion happens too quickly, sugar will enter the bloodstream at a faster rate than the body can handle, sort of like cars getting on the expressway during rush hour. Fortunately, after spending millions of years evolving into the magnificent specimens we are, our bodies have figured out a way to resolve this problem. It involves a hormone secreted by the pancreas, insulin.

The primary job of this biochemical monitor is to regulate blood-sugar levels. Think of insulin as a cop trying to make sure traffic flows smoothly and everybody obeys the speed limit. When all is well, insulin ultimately directs blood sugar to the body's cells where it is stored and used as energy.

However, if blood-sugar conversion is moving too fast, insulin will flip on the sirens, set up roadblocks, chase down, apprehend, and slap the cuffs on every glucose molecule in sight, guilty or not. Then they're carted off to fat-cell jail, fitted for adipose jumpsuits, and put on blood-sugar lockdown. Instead of those just-eaten calories getting a chance to make a productive contribution to your life, they're captured, condemned, and incarcerated, with no chance for community service and/or a normal active life.

What happens next? The streets are empty. Despite the fact that you've just wolfed down a box or two of deep-fried dough, you've got low (or no) blood sugar, so you're left with the inexplicable feeling of a hollow-gut void. This is a false hunger and, girl, a false hunger is the root of all evil. It's also the third most common reason people overeat (the other two follow shortly). Let me break it down.

When a false hunger hits, it's like being single, desperate, and drunk. Yup, that bad. When you're in this state, you're like a junkie—your body doesn't care where it gets sugar from. You'll compromise by eating food you would otherwise never go near, and do some things you would never do in a sober state of mind. One moment you're strolling down the avenue of Self-Control, and the next moment you're standing at the corner of Gotta Have It and Bad Intention, looking for the first cheap treat that comes your way.

Then, before you know it, you're in a quick sugar hook-up getting buzzed from six glazed doughnuts; or you're in a *ménage a trois* doing the wild thing with two pounds of chocolate-covered almonds; or you're trying to wrap your arms around the biggest, greasiest bag of potato chips on the shelf. That's just sad, sad, sad. And while you're moaning and groaning with every chew, in the back of your mind you're thinking, *I hope nobody sees this.* Why? Because it's creating more fat, fat, fat. Then comes the morning after: the insulin hangover and the walk of shame. Just confess to Sister-Self, make things right and head out for a brisk walk.

Rapid carbohydrate conversion can lead to things far worse than a false hunger. A constantly high blood-sugar level can eventually lead to hyperglycemia, which literally means too much sugar. Why is this a problem? Well, check out some of the symptoms and consequences:

- Bad breath (the kind that can melt candle wax)

- Blurred vision (you might not need those glasses and contact lenses after all)

- Dehydration (think dry skin—more scales, wrinkles, and smile lines)

- Dry mouth and chapped lips (no amount of lip gloss in the world will feel soothing)

- Frequent urination (hanging out in the bathroom more than you're living your life?)

- Funky body odor (smells like two cans of fermented pineapple juice)

- Insulin resistance (the packing on of serious mid-body fat)

- Jitteriness and fatigue (the metabolic herky-jerk)

- Poor wound healing (the scab from hell)

- Vaginal itching, rashes, and yeast infections (a big yuck to all of these)

These are all signposts on the road to diabetes. Habitually high blood-sugar levels put a heavy demand and strain on the pancreas to continuously make insulin. Over time, your pancreas is pooped and insulin production *sloooows* down and eventually stops: Exit at insulin resistance, also termed Syndrome X, and welcome to type 2 diabetes. This process, that eventually leads to diabetes, takes approximately two to three years of persistently high blood-sugar (glucose) levels. (*See* Appendix C for additional information on insulin resistance.)

THE GLYCEMIC INDEX

All of this brings us to the all-important glycemic index. *What is this?* you ask. A most excellent question.

The Glycemic Index (GI), developed in 1981 by Dr. David Jenkins and his research team at the University of Toronto, rates how fast a carbohydrate will be converted into sugar and enter your bloodstream after you eat it. These ratings are determined by measuring an individual's glycemic response after eating 50 grams of carbohydrates from a given food source. The higher the GI rating, the faster the blood-sugar conversion rate. The converse is true: the lower on the index, the slower the carbohydrate is converted. Slow is good. Unprocessed carbohydrates, high fiber foods, eaten in the form in which they are grown, are lower. A very high GI is anything above 80 percent, mid-range is 45 to 65 percent, and low is anything under 45 percent. For the glycemic content of common carbohydrate foods, see Table 6.1.

You can pick up a glycemic index reference book at virtually any book-

TABLE 6.1. GLYCEMIC INDEX OF CARBOHYDRATES

Low Glycemic		Moderate	High		
Apples	Greens	Beets	Bagels	Breads:	Alcohol
Asparagus	Kiwi	Brown rice	Banana	whole wheat	Coffee
Broccoli	Peaches	Legumes	Carrots	white (Italian)	(regular
Cauliflower	Pears	Peas	Cereal	Desserts	& decaf)
Citrus	Peppers	Squash	Corn	Low-fat snacks	Soda
Grapes	Plums	Sweet potato	Melon	White potato	(regular
Green beans	Zucchini	Wild rice	Muffins	White rice	& decaf)
			Pasta	White sugar	
10–20%	20–30%	45–65%	80% –	90%	Off the Chart!
GOOD! ⟵			⟶ VERY HIGH		
Thigh Thinning, Insulin Regulating			Fat Storing, Thigh Plumpers		

Note: Healthy PUFA fatty acid foods are under 4%.

store. You could also save a buck or two and just go online and get a list in about twenty seconds. Try to find a list that actually rates brand-name foods, so you can shop more conscientiously. One such list is the *American Journal of Clinical Nutrition* 2002 Glycemic Index. Another is the Revised International Table of Glycemic Index and Glycemic Load Values. (*See* Appendix C and Recommended Reading for additional information on the glycemic index.)

GLYCEMIC LOAD

Glycemic load? I can't slip anything past you. It's not enough, in my opinion, for you to know the GI rating of foods because that number only tells you how quickly a given food will be converted into sugar. What it doesn't tell you is how much carbohydrate is available to be converted from any serving of food, which can dramatically affect blood-sugar levels. In other words, a food can have a high GI but a relatively low carbohydrate total, such as carrots, which are aided by their fiber content. You would have to eat 2–3 cups of carrots to get the same blood-sugar reaction you would have after eating one slice of white, Italian (or most wheat) breads. So go ahead and make like Bugs Bunny. Carrots are cool, eaten in moderation. To lower the GI, you could combine a high GI food with a low GI food. For example, if you combine a carrot (86

GI) with a handful of raw almonds (0 GI), add the two numbers together, and then divide the total by 2, the GI is reduced to a mere 43.

The glycemic load, or GL, is a much better indicator of blood–sugar response than the GI rating alone is, and like the GI rating, the lower the GL, the better. There is an index for this as well, first introduced in 1997 by Dr. Walter Willet and his research team at the Harvard School of Public Health.

A GL above 20 is high, 11–19 is mid-range, and anything under 10 is low. As I mentioned, the international table also gives a glycemic load rating for each food it lists. However, if you can't find the GL for a particular food you're interested in, you can use the following formula to figure it out:

$$(\text{Amount of carbohydrates per serving} \times \text{GI}) \div 100 = \text{GL}$$

For example, one serving of an apple contains 15 grams of carbohydrates and has a GI of 40, and one serving of potatoes has 20 grams of carbohydrates and a GI of 90.

- Apple: $15 \times 40 = 600$; $600 \div 100 = 6$
- Potato: $20 \times 90 = 1{,}800$; $1{,}800 \div 100 = 18$

The apple serving has a low GL of 6 and the potato serving has a mid-range GL of 18, which bolsters the adage: An apple a day keeps the doctor away.

You can make it a lot easier on yourself if you start to think of carbohydrate foods another way. Instead of thinking simple versus complex, think starchy versus filler. Starchy carbohydrate foods contain, well, a lot of starch, which is the actual food made in plants during photosynthesis. Those second grade science lessons are starting to come in handy now, aren't they? Let's jump to the high school level.

Starch is a large organic molecule or polymer (many parts) constructed of many smaller molecules or monomers (one part). When speaking of carbohydrates, the terms polysaccharide (many sugars) and monosaccharide (one sugar) are interchangeable with polymer and monomer, respectively.

Once exposed to digestive enzymes, this gigantic sugar conglomerate of a molecule can be hydrolyzed (broken down) into glucose (a sugar that is used right away) or glycogen (a sugar stored in the muscles or liver). To hydrolyze something simply means to break it apart with water. As you might imagine, starchy carbohydrates (breakfast cereals, corn, potatoes) often have high GI and GL ratings. They pack a load of sugar per serving and, if overly refined and highly processed, are more quickly digested, but yield very few nutrients. The idea then would be to limit your intake of starchy carbohydrates—limit as in cut down on or seriously reduce. This is not the same as eliminate. Some moderate-to-high GL foods have nutritionally redeeming qualities and many really taste good. For me, life totally without hot buttered corn or spuds is not an option. Eat them every day, however, and I'll end up more bovine than divine (I've been accused of being a number of things but a cow is not one of them).

HIGH-FIBER CARBOHYDRATES

High-fiber filler carbohydrates fill you up, which helps with hunger control, as well as blood-sugar regulation. They contain a lot of plant fiber, which can't be hydrolyzed and digested by the body. These plant fibers come in two basic types: insoluble fiber and soluble fiber.

Insoluble Fiber

This type of fiber is made up of plant-cell walls that pass through the digestive tract virtually unchanged. Insoluble fiber helps move food through and regulate the pH (acidity) in your intestines (small and large). Principally found in vegetables, fruits, and their skins, as well as seeds and the bran layer of whole grains, the three main kinds of insoluble fiber are cellulose, hemicellulose, and lignin. Your grandmother called insoluble fiber roughage. Particles of insoluble fiber scrub and clean debris from your arteries, veins, and gastrointestinal tract. They increase peristalsis and activate the colon muscle to move feces and debris out of the body. My favorite saying is, Not only are you *what* you eat, but also what you *don't* excrete!

Soluble Fiber

This type of plant fiber attracts water during digestion and forms a gel, which *sloooows* down the rate at which food enters the small intestine (this keeps it in the stomach longer and results in satiety) and *sloooows* down the rate at which glucose is absorbed into the bloodstream. Principally found in whole grains, such as legumes (beans), in oats, and in raw nuts, the two main kinds of soluble fibers are pectin and gum. Pectin and gum are often used as thickening agents in such foods as ice cream and jellies. These are like a hug from the inside-out foods, making you feel fuller and satiated longer.

Compared to starchy high-glycemic, thigh-swelling carbohydrates, high-fiber filler carbohydrates have lower concentrations of sugar, better GI and GL ratings, and relatively speaking, higher nutritional yields. The idea then would be to choose these types of carbohydrates first. By eating them, you'll also do much to reduce your blood triglyceride and cholesterol levels, because plant fibers are very lipotropic, which means fat-loving. They act as sponges, blotting up gobs of excess lipids and rancid fatty-acid byproducts, which are promptly dispatched via *ye olde* bowel boulevard.

So, if you don't want to buy a book to check the GI and GL ratings, or figure them out for yourself, you could just eat fewer starchy carbohydrates and more filler carbohydrates—fruits and vegetables, in particular.

Here's a tip: Try eating a serving (1 cup or one piece) of fruit or vegetables (better yet, both) at each meal. If you eat smaller feedings every two to three hours, you will have five or six opportunities to get some nutrient-rich, low-glycemic, insulin-friendly, fat-loving plant fibers in your body. Seize the opportunity and redefine your thighs.

So you see, not all carbohydrates are evil as the South Beach or the now-discredited Atkins crusaders and converts would attempt to convince us. However, those refined and highly processed carbohydrates definitely need to be exorcised. Cast out the demons!

Here ends the carbohydrate debate.

Too Fast, Too Much

*H*ow long does it take you to polish off a pork chop? Five minutes? How about a hamburger? Three minutes? What about a slab of ribs? I'm guessing fifteen minutes. What's the rush? The food isn't going anywhere. It's not like you have to kill it and catch it to eat it. It's just lying there on a plate.

Fast eating is the second most common reason people overeat. The faster you eat, the less likely you are to realize that you're full. This is why you have to slow down and chew more. The more you chew, the more you make feel-good satiating chemicals, such as serotonin, dopamine, and CCK (cholecystokinin) that can enter your bloodstream. These neurotransmitters let you know when you've had enough to eat.

Unfortunately, they enter your bloodstream like an eighty-year-old grandmother merging from the on ramp. You have to give them time to drip in and drive home the message that you're satisfied. So, if you try to drive a mini-van of food down your throat at 100 mph—CRASH! BAM! Bye-bye grandma. You're going to overrun your neurotransmitter production and wind up with a serious pile-up on your backside. To avoid this, obey the eating speed limit and—this one's hard to do—attempt to chew at least twenty times before you swallow.

Chewing thoroughly allows for sufficient saturation of neurotransmitters that will let you know when you should get up from the table. Also, the more you chew your food, the more enzymes you expose your food to. Enzymes help break food down, which makes it easier for your stomach to digest and metabolize it. This leads to less gas and better nutrient assimilation, which means you have to eat less to serve your body what it needs. Enzymes are one of the keys to a life of leanness. The slower you eat, the less you will feel the need to eat.

By the way, there are a lot of enzymes in live foods such as legumes, fruits, and vegetables, which is yet another reason you should be eating more of them, daily if possible.

A Couple of Good Tips . . .

- Every time you fill your mouth, put down your fork. This will slow your eating pace down and help break the habit of shoveling up the next forkful before swallowing what's already in your mouth.

- Try ending digestive disruptions while you eat. The less you concentrate on your meal, the more you're stuffing your face. So, stop driving while eating. Stop talking on the phone when you eat. Turn off the TV, too. (I personally pick up a riveting read to slow down my over-zealous consumption time.)

Too Slow, Too Little

*O*K, now it's time to really get in your business. How often are your bowels moving? Yes, I know it's personal but I have to ask. Do you move them every day? Do your feces come out like malt balls or tremendous, tapered torpedoes? Do they feel like labor and delivery when you go, or is it quick-splash, out in a flash? I'm not trying to gross you out, but we have to probe this issue further for reasons you will soon understand.

Your colon, which consists of your large intestine, rectum, and anus, is a $5\frac{1}{2}$ to 6 foot muscular tube about $2\frac{1}{4}$ inches in diameter. Let's get a scope on that. It's longer than the average American woman is tall, is about as big around as two Baby Ruth candy bars held back to back, and could probably outwrestle a sea cucumber. Its primary function is to absorb water, minerals, and nutrients, and to generate and eliminate feces. How much your colon generates and how much it eliminates bring me to my next point.

Wrap a clogged-up colon inside an oversized omentum (remember that word?) and you'll need a boomerang to wrap your belt around your waist. Consider this: The average American woman is walking around with 5–20 pounds of dried, disgusting, crusty, caked-up, preservative-pesticide-parasite-packed, malodorous manure stuck to the walls of her colon. If that doesn't make you want to move your bowels, I don't know what will.

Remember, a healthy bowel's transit time is twelve to twenty-four hours.

47

But the average American woman might take two to three days to expel one meal. If you're not moving it out, you're holding it in, so let's call it what it is, constipation. Americans spend nearly $750 million a year on laxatives. Women suffer from constipation three to four times more than men, so guess who is the primary demographic for these products. You can blame it on eating the chemical nightmare, viral-laden, low-fiber, highly processed, sugar-loaded, highly saturated-transfat foods, no-water-drinking, and, more often than not, a pathetically low-calorie-intake lifestyle that embraces IV-doses of caffeinated libations and overprescribed medications.

Constipation has several consequences, the least of which is having a gut that will make people question when the baby is due. First off, if your colon is backed up, whatever is behind it or in front of it (depending how you look at it) is getting backed up, too. Either way, this means your small intestine. You can't have this happening. Your small intestine is where 90 percent of all the major nutrients enter your bloodstream after they have been broken down into small enough particles to pass through its porous lining.

Here's a good way to think of it. Imagine a window screen with its little holes letting in fresh air. If you smear that screen with a bucket load of colon compost, you'll block up a bunch of those holes and reduce the airflow. The air won't be so fresh anymore, either. Similarly, if your small intestine gets blocked up, you'll reduce your ability to assimilate nutrients. If you're not converting and absorbing nutrients properly, your body will signal you to keep eating until it gets what it needs. Then you're in the catch-22 food snafu: eat more, back up more, assimilate less; crave, eat more, back up more, assimilate less, and crave even more. You could consume food enough to satisfy a sumo wrestler and still be malnourished.

Sister-Self, this is the number-one cause of overeating and constipation.

Lack of enough clean water daily is the third reason people overeat. Plus, water cleans the screen.

Now, you know what it's like to turn on the vacuum cleaner when the bag is full, and how the dirty, dusty debris inside the bag blows back out and gets all over your nice clean furniture and carpet? The same thing happens when you have a stool-packed colon backing up into your small intestine. That foul, fetid, and funky fecal matter you want to so badly be rid of will find its way back into your bloodstream and your blood goes to every cell in your body. Putrid thought, isn't it? Also, the resulting backup pressure forces partially digested large food particles and their toxic metabolites back into your blood. This whole scenario creates dysbiosis, also termed leaky gut syndrome, and it puts your entire body at risk for excessive toxic load. Leaky gut is simply the overgrowth of bad bacteria and excess toxins overtaking the good bacteria in your intestines. It's the beginning of big-time health problems.

If raw sewage is reentering your bloodstream, your body is forced to address this toxic spill problem with some urgency. Imagine if every sink, drainpipe, and toilet in your home started spewing out waste. You'd stop doing whatever you were doing to address that situation, wouldn't you? So, rather than tending to normal metabolic functions, your body becomes pre-occupied with detoxifying itself.

This burdensome task will fall hard on your water-loving kidneys, which will have to work like carnival monkeys on caffeine to keep your system clean. But it will fall like the walls of Jericho on your liver, which filters your blood at a rate of 1.5 quarts a minute. That's 540 gallons a day, and more than 13 million gallons in your lifetime. And if that's not enough, your liver also has to:

- Break down insulin and other hormones
- Make glucose
- Manufacture and process cholesterol
- Process medicines and toxic by-products
- Produce bile (can't digest or absorb fat without it)
- Regulate blood clotting
- Store vitamins and minerals
- Synthesize folic acid—and if you're pregnant, make red blood cells for your fetus during its first three months of existence

Just because your liver is the largest organ in your body doesn't mean it wants to work that hard all the time. So, please, for your liver's sake, try to clean up your act a bit.

Do you remember the pH scale? You probably learned about it in the third grade. It measures the acidity and alkalinity of a substance on a scale from 1–14, with 1 being most acidic and 14 being most alkaline (base). Water is considered neutral with a pH of 7. The body fluids of really healthy people fall into a pH range of 7–7.5, while your blood absolutely, positively has to maintain a pH of 7.4. If it fluctuates up or down by one-tenth of a point—red lights and sirens—you're off to the intensive care unit. If it moves by two-tenths of a point—black dresses and organ music—call the undertaker.

Now, when your colon starts giving you a lot of attitude and gets all funky on you and clams up, your body is headed for pH jeopardy.

So, what's going on or not going on in your colon represents the single biggest threat to your health. Your colon is the foundation of your house. If it's leaking, blocked, or backed up, it poses a threat to every cell in your body. All diseases begin at the cellular level, with the colon considered to be at the foundation of good health. Unfortunately for backed-up colons, there are scores of illnesses and ailments related to colon toxicity and hyperacidity. Consider a few:

- Abdominal distension (putrefying stools, make a lot of gas, which blows up your colon like a balloon)
- Acid reflux
- Arthritis (large food particles in the bloodstream can cause joint inflammation)
- Asthma
- Backaches
- Breast cancer
- Colorectal cancer (second only to breast cancer as the leading cancer killer of women in America)
- Chronic fatigue
- Crohn's disease
- Diabetes
- Diverticulitis
- Endometriosis
- Estrogen reabsorption, which increases your risk for tender breasts and a toxic lymph system
- Food allergies (your immune system will attack large food particles as foreign pathogens)
- Fibromyalgia
- Flatulence (the deadly kind that makes you afraid to sneeze in the elevator)

- Gray hair
- Halitosis and foul body odor (if you think you're lonely now)
- Headaches
- Hemorrhoids
- High cholesterol
- Hypertension
- Hypoglycemia
- Insomnia
- Infertility
- Irritable bowel syndrome
- Irritability (you can't be happy with constipation and the piles)
- Overactive bladder (it will dribble increasingly with a compacted colon bearing down on it)
- Polyps
- Premature aging
- Recurrent sinusitis (the more toxic you are, the more mucous your body will make to trap the toxins)
- Reproductive tissue cysts
- Sciatic pain (the nerve runs right under the intestinal tract)
- Skin irritations
- Spastic colon
- Ulcerative colitis
- Weight gain
- Yeast infections

A lot of things can run afoul in the bowel. Now, let me tell you what to do about this.

WATER

You can't flush a toilet without it, right? If there's no water in your colon, how is it going to flush the stool out? Besides, your body is approximately 60 to 65 percent water. If you were to be vacuum-dried, you could fit into a shoebox.

If you don't give your body the elements it's primarily made of, how do you expect it to function properly? And if it doesn't function properly, it will *sloooow* down. If it *sloooows* down, your metabolism *sloooows* down, and you get fat. See the connection?

You have to drink water. I didn't say fluids. I said water. Coffee, juice, milk shakes, soda, tea, beer and wine—that stuff doesn't count. They all need water to be digested, so drinking them only dehydrates you more. Call it a bottle of Fiji, Crystal Geyser, or Trinity, call it a Lake Michigan cocktail, call it tap, fountain, or hose—just drink it. However, avoid mineral-deficient dis-tilled water, ideal for irons and fountains only.

Get this. If you don't drink enough water, your body will discreetly secrete a hormone called aldosterone that will actually force your body to retain more of it. Yeah, no kidding. You can get bloated if you don't drink enough water. Truth is stranger than fiction, isn't it?

With a neutral pH of 7, water is your best defense against toxicity and your best prevention against acidity. It is also the most vital stimulant for peri-stalsis, the wavelike undulating movement of the colon that actually pushes the stools out of the chute. The truth be known, dehydration is the greatest cause of constipation, not poor fiber intake (a very close second, though).

Now, for the question of the ages: How much water do you need to drink every day? The standard line has always been to drink eight glasses a day. But what does that really mean? A glass could be 4 ounces, 10 ounces, or 16 ounces, and a Big Gulp at 7-Eleven is close to half a gallon. I've got some-thing to help you here. Try this formula I use to calculate water intake for my clients:

Weight $\times$ .075 = total daily cups of water needed per day
Note: 1 cup = 8 ounces

Following this formula, the average American woman's daily water need is:

143 $\times$ .075 = 10.72 cups
Or: 10.72 cups $\times$ 8 ounces per cup = 85.8 ounces

With water, as with most nutrients, there is a supply and demand consid-eration. You may need more water, which could depend on whether or not you're:

• In a hot climate or environment for an extended period

• Involved in strenuous physical activity or exercise for any protracted state

• Recovering from an injury or illness

• Under great stress

For any of these you might consider a hydration ratio of 1 ounce of water per pound of body weight.

Calculate the amount of water your body needs for what it must do. It might take you some time to adjust to the increase, but work up slowly, cup by cup, week by week, until you reach your optimal amount. Stay steady in your increased consumption throughout the day or you will be in the bathroom more than you

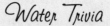

Water Trivia

If you find you're urinating non-stop, after three to four weeks add a multimineral to your daily agenda. Take two, 3 times a day after each meal. This helps move water into the kidney cells, decreasing excessive urination.

will be living your life. Your colon will be most grateful, and so will your hips, thighs, and waist. You'll also have clearer skin and fewer wrinkles. Compare a water-filled grape to a raisin and you'll see what I mean. Every screen siren, video vixen, and catwalk cover girl worth her weight in diamonds knows that water is her best beauty aid. And drinking it keeps you cool, literally. (*See* Appendix B for additional information on water.)

FIBER

You know that your colon is $5\frac{1}{2}$ to 6 feet long. Add to that your small intestine, all 20 to 22 feet of it, and that's a lot of plumbing. You need something to push the food and stools through that amount of tubing. That's why, for lovely thighs you have to eat fiber, at least 25–30 grams a day.

By comparison, most Americans consume less than 8 grams a day. To give you an idea of what the daily fiber recommendation translates into, one medium apple contains approximately 2–3 grams. So, if you don't want to eat ten to sixteen apples a day, start exploring the vast and varied, delicious and delectable wonderland of fruits, vegetables, legumes, and lastly organic whole grains, which have the unprocessed, nutrient-dense bran contained within them (that's why they're called whole).

You might also want to consider taking a fiber supplement because consuming 25–30 grams of fiber is no small task. Make sure it's a fiber supplement, though, and not a laxative. Laxatives just liquefy your stool. Take enough of them long enough and you'll end up with a lazy colon that forgets what it's supposed to do. Laxatives also flush and deplete you of vital minerals, which can lead to serious dehydration and electrolyte imbalances—we're talking angina, dizziness, headaches, heart attacks, and muscle cramps, if you overdo it. You do not have to abuse your bowels to have a seemingly respectable bowel movement.

Eating more fiber also means drinking more water. This insoluble fiber can absorb as much as ten times its weight in water. Soluble fiber can absorb 40, 60, even 200 times its weight in water. If you don't get enough water into your intestinal track, whatever fiber you're eating is going to have the opposite effect of constipating you. Think intestinal fur balls. Again, just drink enough water.

An intake of 50-percent soluble and 50-percent insoluble fiber is ideal, but don't stress out about it. If you're having hearty bowel movements (18 inches to 24 inches) but still experience appetite control problems, eat more soluble fiber foods and healthy fat–based foods, such as avocados, hummus, raw nut butters, and nuts (not peanut butter!). If your appetite is under control and you're having poor bowel movements, you need to eat more of the low-glycemic, starchy, carbohydrate-based foods, and most likely need to increase your intake of both water and healthy fatty-acid foods. See how easy that is? FYI: Flaxseed is a perfect fifty-fifty blend of the two types of fiber.

Realize that a $5\frac{1}{2}$-foot colon is 66 inches long. Ideally, you would like your food to make a complete run through your colon, from cecum to rectum, every two to three days. So, you should be excreting a minimum of 22 inches of intact stool, 3 inches in diameter, daily.

The average American woman generally doesn't excrete even 8–10 inches of broken-up stool in two to three days. You should be able to do this without straining, as straining can lead to hemorrhoids. Your stool should be soft, but formed, three fingers wide in diameter (a clogged colon makes skinny stools) and light to medium brown in color (dark brown means not enough fiber; black can mean blood, requiring that you see a doctor). And the scent should not chase the dog out of the house.

Before we move on, let me ask you a question related to all of this. Have you ever done a detox? No, I'm not talking about drug rehab. I don't know if you know this or not, but pesticides, preservatives, pollutants, and pharma-

Helpful Trivia

- **Bonus trivia:** The fiber and enzymes in fruits and vegetables also act like a scrub brush and detergent. They help keep your small intestine screen open (good nutrient assimilation) and your colon crud-free (less weight, less toxicity).

- **Double bonus trivia:** Your colon supports more than sixty different kinds of beneficial bacteria (acidophilus, bifidus, and *Saccharomyces boulardii* are three of the most beneficial). All help nutrient assimilation, maintain normal pH, and fight viruses, bad bacteria overgrowth, fungus (*Candida albicans,* the dreaded yeast, for example), plus parasitic colonization. Fruits and vegetables help maintain a healthy microflora (bacterial composition) throughout your intestinal tract.

FYI: Florastor is the perfect intestinal villi rebuilder.

- **Triple bonus trivia:** Foods rich in plant fiber are also called negative-calorie foods because they force your body to burn more calories during digestion than they actually yield. Eat them and not only will you keep your colon clean, you'll enhance your nutrient uptake, feel full, control your weight, and burn calories, all at the same time. Wow!

ceuticals are all chemicals, and chemicals have what's called a half-life. Now, a half-life can be defined in one or two ways, but essentially both meanings are the same:

1. A half-life is the time required for a radioactive substance to lose 50 percent of its activity through decay. (For example, plutonium-239 has a half-life of 24,000 years.) You may not have much contact with radon, but you are probably breathing in some wherever you are. Radon is a radioactive gas released by the uranium found in soil and rocks under or near a lot of

homes. It has a half-life of four days. Now, if you're always breathing it in, radon has a longer life within you.

2. A half-life is the time required for the level of a substance in the body (drug, toxin, pollutant) to have 50 percent of its concentration reduced through elimination from the body.

As you can see, the amount of time these toxins spend in your body can be anywhere from days to a lifetime of years. Frightening thought, isn't it? So, to insure that your bloodstream and plumbing system are clear and clean, consider doing a biannual detox. Think of it as fall- and spring-cleaning. There are many products available for this purpose. However, a two-to-four-day live and green juice fast works quite well, provided the juice is fresh squeezed and is not the pasteurized, sugar-spiked kind from a bottle or a carton. Though pasteurization kills the bacteria that can cause spoilage, making for a longer shelf life, it also makes the juice less nutritious and more acidic.

It wouldn't hurt to get a colonic every now and then, either. Despite your best efforts, fecal and mucous plaque still build up on the walls of your colon. Also, if you have long endured constipation and irregular bowel movements, a series of colonics may help rid you of a bad intestinal history. My daughter, Christina (I love her dearly), is the chief colon hydrotherapist and educator at our center. She once had a client in her mid-thirties who discharged a large wad of putrefied meat during a treatment. Yep, it just came flying right out of her. Stop laughing. This individual had been a vegetarian for five years. Kind of makes you wonder what's hanging around in your colon, hmm?

One more thing: Listen to Katie Couric and get a colonoscopy every eight to ten years. A congested colon can present more than a heavy-duty booty and a tubby tummy. In America, one person dies from colorectal cancer every 9.3 minutes. That's almost 155 people a day and nearly 57,000 people a year. Clean it up, clear it out, stay alive, and live well and long. (*See* Appendix F for additional information on colonics.)

Now, let's go from cleaning colons to dietary design.

Pyramids Are for Building

The Great Pyramid of Giza is one of the Seven Wonders of the World. It was built by the Egyptians almost 5,000 years ago and it weighs more than 6 million tons. That's impressive.

Maybe this is the reason the United States Department of Agriculture (USDA) decided to use the pyramid as a model for how we should eat. I'm guessing they were on a field trip in Cairo when they had this dietary moment of inspiration.

One year after Operation Desert Storm began in 1991, the USDA decided to release its new weapon in the war on nutritional ambiguity. They hired the American Dietetic Association (ADA) to turn the four-food-groups, balanced-diet concept, originally developed in the 1950s, into a convenient symbol—the food pyramid. This was supposed to help us all eat healthier and lose weight faster than you could say Tutankhamen.

Time out. Let's go back to the beginning of this section for a quick review. Pyramids are little on the top and enormously huge on the bottom, right? They tip the scales at an ungodly amount of weight, right? And they maintain their structure for a long, long, long time, right? Does this sound like something you want to emulate?

My rationale is this: If you eat like the pyramid, you'll look like the pyramid—small on top and large on bottom, with thunder thighs. Follow the

USDA's modern wonder of the world and a team of archeologists might come prospecting on your behind one day, looking for the remains of an ancient Egyptian pharaoh.

Almost since its debut in 1992, this icon of *myth* conception has been assailed by every rational, objective, scientific evaluator who can read. No less than Dr. Walter Willett (yep, same guy who gave us the Glycemic Load Index) said in his book, *Eat, Drink, and Be Healthy,* "At best, the USDA pyramid offers wishy-washy, scientifically unfounded advice on an absolutely vital topic—what to eat."

Ouch. That had to hurt. Fourteen years later, both the U.S. Surgeon General and the Centers for Disease Control (CDC) confirm Dr. Willet's criticism: 65 percent of adults, that's more than 130 million Americans, are overweight or obese. Coincidence? I think not.

The ADA endorses eating eleven servings of carbohydrates a day, as the foundation of its nutritional polyhedron. It does this without glycemic distinction, essentially declaring that all carbohydrates are not only equal but good for us, too. I know, and you know, this isn't true. All carbohydrates are not equal in nutrient profile, fiber composition, or glycemic reaction. While some are nutritionally noble, others are downright fat-forming and thigh-dimpling.

Likewise, the food pyramid wrongly lumps all fats into one class and categorically deems them as being bad. That's just as wrong—basically, it's a big fat lie. In a June 13, 2002, article in the *Wall Street Journal,* Dr. Willet stated, "The pyramid really ignored 40 years of data and condemned all fats and oils."

Dr. Willet's colleague at the Harvard School of Public Health, Dr. Frank Hu, offered a similar critique about the disinformation disservice the food pyramid promotes for protein. In the August 2004 issue of *Men's Fitness* magazine, Dr. Hu opined, "According to the pyramid, all protein sources offer the same nutritional benefits, but we know that's no longer true . . . The food pyramid also says we should think of all sources of protein and carbohydrates as being the same, but in today's world, we just can't do that anymore."

Case in point. On the pyramid, legumes, meats, and nuts are shelved in the same category. Also, plant protein is considered the same as animal protein. Now, a rib-eye steak may have fewer calories per gram of protein than, say, a bowl of pinto beans. But that bowl of beans has the type of dietary fiber (steak contains no fiber) that will keep your colon clear and soak up some of the saturated fat from that steak, lowering your cholesterol. Dairy products, another source of protein, contain conjugated linoleic acid, which helps metabolize fats and proteins. However, since dairy is considered the number-one allergy food, I suggest black currant-seed oil, borage, or pure evening primrose oil as supplements. Nuts are rich in vitamin E, which helps lower the risk of diabetes, heart disease, and strokes and counters the development of cataracts. Coldwater fish is busting at the gills with omega-3 fatty acids, which improve vascular health and help alleviate the symptoms of rheumatoid arthritis and psoriasis, while improving insulin sensitivity. How can all of these foods be treated as equal sources of protein, offering the same nutritional benefits? They can't.

Many things about both the USDA and the ADA dietary monument crinkle my brow, but one thing, more than any other, just baffles, befuddles, and bewilders me to no end: Nowhere is there any mention of water.

Hellooooo, water is the source of life. It covers 70 percent of the planet. It's the most abundant natural resource. And at birth, 70-plus percent of your body is water, for crying out loud. Think about this. Have you ever heard of people going on hunger strikes? Yes, you have. You can go for weeks without eating solid food and survive. Now, have you ever heard of people going on water strikes? No, you haven't. You'd need a friggin' miracle to stay alive for more than four days without water. How can a nutrition guide developed and promoted by the USDA, as the authority for how we are to eat, not mention water? Unbelievable.

Here's the real kicker. The USDA and the ADA came out with a revised version of the food pyramid on April 19, 2005, and *still* left water out of the pyramid. You'd think, after thirteen years, somebody, anybody involved with this venerable vanguard of public health would have considered adding the most important thing you could put in your mouth to its own "guide for healthy living" pyramid. And speaking of thirteen years, by law, nutritional guidelines are supposed to be revised every five years. I wonder if being eight years late counts as some sort of violation?

By the way, the new food pyramid is now called My Pyramid. This sounds like something you order across the counter at a fast-food joint. Whoa—talk about karmic coincidence. Just as this new nutritional model was being introduced to the world, McDonald's was offering fifty-cent cheeseburgers to celebrate its fiftieth birthday. Now, that's timing.

Michael Johanns, Secretary of the USDA, boasts that My Pyramid was designed to stress a more personalized approach to better health. This geometric, got-it-wrong-again pyramid is a vertical rainbow, with a runner scaling a flight of stairs—that's to promote exercise, which is the best thing about the new My Pyramid.

First of all, to be literal about it (as I was with the pyramid's shape), everyone knows that rainbows arc across the sky and are not vertical. If you ever start seeing rainbows that go straight up and down, you'll know that the end times are near. Secondly, if you eat the way this latest pyramid tells you to, you definitely will not be able to run up a flight of stairs.

On April 20, 2005, just one day after the USDA unveiled this mealtime marvel, Margo G. Wootan, Nutritional Policy Director for the Center for Science in the Public Interest, had this to say about it on www.consumer affairs.com: "This new symbol is a missed opportunity. The USDA and the ADA seem to have bent over backwards to avoid upsetting any particular commodity group or food company by not showing any foods that Americans should eat less of . . . There are simple key principles about healthy eating that truly do work for all Americans, and those could have been represented on one symbol."

I could not have said it better myself. In Director Wootan's statement lie clues that offer insight into the inadequacies of the food pyramid. It contains the words *upsetting, commodity,* and *food company.* You have to ask yourself, who are the benefactors of the ADA? Could it possibly be junk food manufacturers?

The very first food pyramid was scheduled to make its public debut in April of 1991. Its initial design was intended to promote a greater consumption of grains, fruits, and vegetables, while encouraging a lower consumption of diary products and meats. This didn't sit well with the beef and dairy lobbyists who had a cow-mooing, bull-snorting fit over a government-sponsored campaign that would cut into their profits. After a bit of cud-chewing and horn-ramming, the pyramid was refined and revealed a year later.

Politics—they're everywhere, even in our supposedly healthy food guides. Countless special interest groups—beef brokers, dairy dealers, grain growers, pork purveyors, poultry peddlers, sugar suppliers, and agricultural agents of every type—are all lobbying for the coveted big-base bottom spot. Whoever gets that spot stands to make a pharaoh's ransom from the copious consumer consumption of its goods. This is, in part, why the revised model went from horizontal blocks to vertical stripes, in an attempt to appease the multifaceted, me-first food manufacturers and merchants of America.

Consequently, many critics, myself included, are very suspicious of any food model put forth by the ADA and endorsed by the USDA, as it weighs the pressures and greediness of the food industry against the sound principles needed to develop a healthy eating strategy for the nation. There, I said it.

Aside from the water oversight, neither the old or new pyramid ever effectively addressed what is perhaps most responsible for the sidewalk-cracking tonnage of our citizenry. Interested?

Attention all blood-pumping Americans: Whether you live in a red state or a blue state, whether you like Bill O'Reilly and Alan Colmes or Al Franken and Jon Stewart, you need to understand something: **Junk food is the crack cocaine of nutrition**.

No question about it, junk food is hard to resist. The lure of all that fat, salt, and sugar is overpowering. The artificial flavors and colors conceal its potency, but all it takes is one munch, one crunch, one dip, one sip, and you could be hooked forever.

It starts when you're a kid, with the corn-sugar-laden juices, the lollipops, and the cookies. Soon afterward, you're into the hard stuff: Ho-Hos, Rolos, Cheetos, Oreos, Klondikes, Mike and Ikes, Paydays, Frito Lays. That's when the jonesing starts, those addict-habit cravings that always have you fixated on the next fix. Then, years later, you wake up one morning in a dorm room and realize you can't brush your teeth without downing a liter of Mountain Dew first. The blood-sugar desperation becomes more frequent because the more junk you eat, the more junk you need to get that junk-food high. Your blood sugar goes up, down, and round and round.

Just picture it: Your once lean thighs are trembling and your hands are shaking because your glucose levels have hit rock bottom. You're scouring the streets looking for a Butterfinger like a crackhead on a three-day binge. Before long, your name is a regular on the blubber blotter. Street-corner camera footage of you hitting every convenience store in town will be gathered daily, and you'll wind up with a diabetic rap sheet as wide as your behind. Your life will be filled with empty wrappers and useless calories, and you'll be headed for cardiac hell.

Heed the truth in the humor because the addiction to junk food is no joke, and the junk-food pushers know this. They count on it, spending more than $33 billion a year marketing their version of addictive narcotics to us. In exchange, we dish out more than $120 billion buying their products. Plump return on their investment, I say.

However, we pay a far greater cost. According to the CDC's own statistics, 18.2 million Americans have diabetes, and a third of them don't even know it; it's the sixth-leading cause of death, killing more than 200,000 people every year. Medical and related costs total more than $130 billion annually.

More than 1.4 million new cases of nonsmoking, nonskin-related cancers arise each year; it's the second leading cause of death, claiming in excess of 570,000 lives every January through December, or 1,500 lives each day; medical and related costs are equal to more than $69 billion annually.

Upward of 70 million people, more than one-quarter of the population, have some form of heart disease; it continues as the leading cause of deaths, killing more than 927,000 people a year, or one person every thirty-four seconds. Medical and related costs total more than $394 billion annually.

Diseases related to obesity and being overweight wipe out more than 112,000 lives every year; medical and related spending is more than $117 billion annually.

Consider this intervention done. I'm a realist and I know that America is not ever likely to totally purge this junk-food scourge from our eating habits. On a more personal note, having already become addicted to junk foods makes your chance of giving it up completely extremely difficult. If you can escape the junk-food habit, great, but if you can't, all is not lost.

In many ways, we are a nation of intoxication, so my recommendation is moderation—moderation, moderation, moderation is the way. But that does not mean every single day.

All right, enough fire and brimstone. What I'm going to lay on you next is quite radical. Some in the nutrition world might even say heretical. Hold on to your broccoli.

The food pyramid, as you now know, had its origins with the four basic food groups, which are:

1. Fruits and vegetables

2. Breads and cereals

3. Protein foods

4. Dairy foods

Here's where it gets controversial. There aren't four food groups. There never were. There are, and always have been, only two food groups: physical health food and mental health food.

You eat to be healthy and you eat to be happy. Brussels sprouts, navel oranges, pomegranate juice, and free-roaming, skinless, hormone-free chicken breasts make you healthy. Cheeseburgers, cherry turnovers, French fries, and piña coladas make you happy. Now, if you're only eating to be healthy, you're going to miss out on some mighty tasty happiness. If you're only eating to be happy, you're going to blow your shot at being healthy.

I have met some wheat-grass, granola-crunching, free-range-eating people with 0-percent body fat who are as miserable as a stepped-on bunion. And I have met some ice-cream, double-layer-cake, butter-on-everything people who are as sweet as what they eat, but a heartbeat shy of a triple bypass. Living life to either extreme seems undesirable to me.

But this isn't an all-or-nothing scenario. You want to be happy and healthy, so the key is balancing your intake of these two food groups. You need more physical health food than you need mental health food to stay alive, healthy, and lean. Staying alive is a priority. If you're not alive and healthy, happy has zero chance for existence.

You need less mental health food than you need physical health food because happy food feeds your moods. If you are always in the mood for happy food, and never in the mood for healthy food, then, as I said earlier, you have other appetites that aren't being met. That's a point of personal exami-

Sweet-Treat Tip

If you do a sweet treat, don't do a cheap treat. Cheap treats are a dime a dozen. You can buy a package of cookies at the supermarket and wolf down enough calories to fuel Lance Armstrong through one leg of the Tour de France. On the other hand, you could take the same amount of money and spend it on a delicious, gourmet-quality chocolate truffle and only eat about one-twentieth the amount of calories. After all, a treat is just that, a treat. It isn't a meal. If you're hungry, feed your body not your mood. Got it? Good.

nation you need to tend to with all due speed—ignoring your mind, body, or spiritual well-being could adversely affect all levels of your health.

While on the subject of balancing food groups, I want to put this whole balanced-diet thing in perspective and discuss nutrient balance. First of all, do you really know what a nutrient is? That may seem like a strange question at this point in the book. I just think it's important to be fully aware of words when we use them, and most people aren't. Try to define trust—quickly, quickly, GONG! You see, it's not so easy.

So, for the sake of clarity: A nutrient is any substance vital for life functions and growth. Easy enough. For our purposes, these substances include carbohydrates, fats, proteins, water, vitamins, and minerals. Some people also

Trivia Time

Did you know that chocolate contains a natural substance called phenylethylamine? It stimulates the same chemical reaction in your body that occurs when you fall in love. Kind of gives a whole new meaning to chocoholic. When you say, *I love chocolate,* most likely you really mean it.

define a nutrient by its calorie content and thus include alcohol, which not only has a high-caloric carbohydrate yield but, alas, is very high on the glycemic index. I suspect these people have self-serving motives at play, given that water, the most vital of all nutrients, has no calories, and alcohol certainly can't be considered vital for life functions and growth. I have, however, seen times when a robust glass of red wine was essential to my mental health by week's end.

Moderation . . . moderation . . . moderation is the way.

So far, we've covered carbohydrates and water reasonably well but have merely alluded to the others. How about a quick breakdown on what they are and how much of them we need?

PROTEIN

Protein is a highly complex nitrogenous (contains nitrogen) molecule made up of one or more amino-acid chains. An amino acid is a smaller molecule made from an amino group (nitrogen, hydrogen) and a carboxylic group (carbon, oxygen, and hydrogen). Don't get caught up on the super scientific terminology. You're not going to get tested on this later.

There are literally hundreds of amino acids that exist in nature, but there are only twenty-two that are important to human nutrition. Fourteen of these can be manufactured by the body and are called non-essential. For adults, eight must be obtained from food sources (nine for babies) and are called essential. Just as amino acids are often referred to as the building blocks of protein, proteins are often referred to as the building blocks of the body. Nice symmetry there. Protein yields 4 calories per gram and is extremely important for you to eat. Ponder its many functions, as seen in the inset on the following page.

Just as amino acids can be classified as non-essential and essential, proteins are similarly classified as complete or incomplete. If a protein source contains high amounts of all the essential amino acids, all nine, then it is considered complete. Egg, animal, and fish protein are examples. Incomplete protein sources lack one or more essential amino acids of which legumes, nuts, seeds, and leafy vegetables are examples. That is why you should eat your beans with rice. Together, they contain the essential amino acids needed

Functions of Protein

- Activates adrenal and thyroid support
- Builds and re-oxygenates tissue
- Forms neurotransmitters
- Generates muscle energy (ATP)
- Helps manufacture the building blocks that assist in making 500-plus regulatory hormones daily
- Develops the backbone for a strong immune system and glandular functions
- Helps in enzyme production
- Increases vitamin and mineral absorption
- Maintains healthy ovarian function
- Processes and transports fat

- Produces antibodies
- Produces hormones, such as insulin
- Regulates blood sugar and maintains proper glucose levels (appetite control)
- Regulates the endocrine (glandular) system
- Regulates the pancreas and insulin production
- Regulates the pineal gland, often termed the enlightenment gland, or your third eye
- Synthesizes the myelin sheath (protective covering) for nerve cells
- Transports oxygen

Note: Protein is the main ingredient in skin (collagen, elastin), hair and nails (keratin), and muscles (myosin).

to make a complete protein. Ah-hah. (*See* Appendix D for additional information on amino acids.)

Highly bioavailable proteins are lean, less contaminated, and contain a higher ratio of vitamins and minerals. These include wild coldwater fish, humanely treated and killed, nonhormone-laden, pesticide-free, organically fed, happy, truly free-range poultry, loin cuts of beef, lamb, and pork. Low bioavailability is generally found in bacon, fast-food meats, hot dogs, luncheon meats, and salami, as well as meats sourced from highly stressed caged animals. You are what you eat.

Most women are notoriously pathetic protein eaters, while many men will eat the entire backside of a cow in one sitting. Women will eat half a turkey sandwich at lunch and call it a day.

An Alarming Insight

If you don't consume enough protein, your body will take protein from its own tissue—the most expendable source first: your skin. So, if you don't want to look fifty-five when you're forty, consume high-quality bioavailable protein sources at breakfast, lunch, and dinner.

It's now time to figure out how much protein you need every day. The standard line is 1 gram for every two pounds of body weight. For the average 143-pound American woman, this would mean a daily intake of 71.5 grams (143 pounds ÷ 2), which has an energy value of 497 calories. If you use the 1,716-calorie (weight × 12) daily-intake value previously determined, her protein total would represent nearly 30 percent of her daily caloric intake. You're going to be teaching math at NASA before this book is done.

Though this ratio serves most people well enough, there are other ratios to consider, such as those based on lifestyle and activity demands.

Sedentary to Moderately Active

Take moderately active to mean twenty to thirty minutes of exercise two to four days a week. For the average American woman, that's 57.2 grams a day, which is roughly 399 calories, or about 23 percent of her daily caloric intake.

Active

This is for the person who engages in forty-five to sixty minutes of hearty exercise five to six days a week. For the average American woman, that's a range of 85.8–100.1 grams a day, which is about 595 calories, or 35 percent of her daily caloric intake.

Highly Active

Think intense physical laborer, highly conditioned athlete, bodybuilder, or someone recovering from serious illness or surgery. For the average American woman on approximately 2,000 calories a day, that's a range of 85–110 grams a day, which is about 650–785 calories, or approximately 35 percent of her daily caloric intake.

Note: If dealing with, or recovering from, a long-term illness, surgery, chemotherapy, or radiation, use the highly active formula to calculate protein requirements.

I tend to make recommendations based on 30 percent of daily caloric intake rather than a grams-to-body weight ratio. I find this calculation more serviceable when combining an optimal nutritional intake with the amount conducive for appetite satiation and cellular regeneration. I suggest a protein intake that is 28 to 30 percent of your daily caloric intake. For the average nonexercising American woman who is consuming 1,200 calories a day, this means a calorie count of 360 calories from protein and a total of 50–55 grams. (*See* Appendix G for information on daily food logs and *"Protein ounce to gram"* explanation.)

Your body can't store extra protein, so if you take in too much, the excess will either be used as excess energy, if needed, or stored as fat. Also, bear in mind that the most protein you can digest and assimilate at one sitting is 28–32 grams, the equivalent of four eggs or 4.5 ounces of chicken. Those 48-ounce porterhouse steaks some restaurants serve are beyond stupid and absurd. Talk about a sledgehammer to your pancreas. You would have to be a jungle carnivore to handle that much protein at one meal. Oh, and protein puts a big water demand on the body. Your body requires twice as much water to metabolize protein versus carbohydrates. Again, drink it.

Good Tips

- If you want to increase absorbency with your protein intake, consider using a whey-based protein powder. Whey is the single most compatible form of protein for the body. It makes up about 70 percent of the protein in human breast milk. It is high in immunoglobulins that are cancer fighters. Powders list the exact gram amount per serving on the container, so you know precisely what you're ingesting. Whey isolate protein powder is best.

- You can find precise values in certain protein bars, too, but be mindful of what protein source is used in them as well as the total amount of sugar (they should be under 4 grams). Most important, avoid any bar that contains hydrogenated or trans fats and preservatives. A good protein bar will contain fiber and healthy fat.

FATS

I started to give you a definition for this in the Preface. Just for the record, fat is a three-carbon chain glycerol (hence the term triglyceride) that bonds to a carboxylic group (remember the amino acid combination?) via oxygen. Short and sweet. Got it? Good. Now make like the Sopranos and fuhgeddaboudit.

All you need to remember is that your body absolutely needs good fats. I know what you've heard—that all fats are bad and therefore bad for you. Not true. That low-fat-mantra originated in the 1960s, followed by the slam-dunk high-carbohydrate craze of the 1990s. You can thank the food pyramid of 1991 for the hysteria. Yup, that thing again. Somebody get a hammer.

Fat became the new three-letter word and a big no-no to eat. Funny thing though, while a Salem witch-hunt for any food with fat in it was going on, people were scaling new heights in obesity. That doesn't make sense. How could this happen? Fat-free food, that's how. Thinking they were OK to eat,

NEWS FLASH

Fat-free doesn't mean calorie-free. All those
extra carbohydrates that were once praised
as nutritional saints became fat converters.
Lesson learned.

people were overdosing on high-sugar, high-carbohydrate, fake fat foods that
were totally devoid of nutrients.

This will blow your mind. For the last 100,000 years (90,000 of which
people spent as hunter-gatherers) the hormone profile and metabolism of
humans has remained virtually unchanged. The significance of this is that
grains and the subsequently processed carbohydrate foods they became
(breads, crackers, pastas, among others) have only been a steady part of our
diet since the advent of agriculture. What's my point? Simply that our bodies
are far better equipped and suited to handle fats than carbohydrates.
WHAMMO . . . I'll bet that hit you right between the eyes.

Yep, long before we ever contemplated dumplings, matzo balls, and
pierogies, people were satiated by, and learned to proficiently digest, the fats
and oils from momma's milk, animals, eggs, nuts, and seeds. When people
started with milk formulas, scooping up gnocchi, and eating Wonder bread,
they started getting ear and yeast infections, insulin resistance, diabetes, and
so on. Eons ago, when people ate fat, they used it. Today, not so well. Skip
ahead to the Marathon-candy era, enter the world of fake fats; pack in the
high sugar and store more and more . . . fat that is.

You already know that fat is a long-term energy fuel yielding 9 calories
per gram, and that it is stored in places you would rather not discuss. But did
you know about all the many incredible things healthy fats do for, and inside
of, your body? See the inset on the following page for more on fat.

Some fats, such as phospholipids (these form cell membranes and transport other fats around), prostaglandins (anti-inflammatory agents), and
steroids, as well as wax (stick a Q-tip in your ear), are made by the body.
Other needed fats are obtained by ingesting them—hence the term essential

Functions of Fat

- Adds form to killer curves
- Aids in blood clotting
- Decreases inflammation
- Delays hunger pangs
- Enhances vaginal, joint, and eye lubrication
- Helps with the absorption of vitamins and minerals
- Influences blood pressure (vasodilation and vasoconstriction)
- Insulates the body
- Aids in circulation
- Keeps skin supple
- Keeps *ye olde* stool chute slip-sliding (no straining means no hemorrhoids and that's a relief)
- Activates thyroid, regulates body temperature
- Makes hair shiny and thick
- Mitigates glucose spikes
- Prevents brittle nails
- Protects vital organs from impact
- Provides cushion for bones
- Provides satiety
- Reduces carbohydrate cravings
- Regulates menstruation (lack of fat can lead to amenorrhea) involved in the synthesis of hormones
- Stimulates smooth muscle tissue
- Builder of all hormones and neurotransmitters

fatty acids (EFAs). These are called omega-3s and omega-6s, both fatty acids high in wondrous linoleic acid. Thankfully, these can be found in many food sources and it's best to eat a variety. (*See* Appendix A for additional information on essential fatty acids.)

Nature's fats come in three physical states—saturated fats, polyunsaturated fats, and monounsaturated fats—each of which will be discussed below, along with hydrogenated fats.

Saturated Fats

Saturated fats are solid at room temperature and are primarily found in meat and dairy products like butter (*yummm*). Palm and coconut oil also fall in this category. With the exception of coconut butter—high in lauric acid, a good-for-you medium-chain fatty acid that does not enhance your fat stores readily. This good guy, normalizes high cholesterol, protects your liver, reduces inflammation, and actually helps burn stored hazardous saturated fats—these are the fats to watch out for because they stick to the walls of your blood vessels, clog up your heart valves, jack up your bad LDL and cholesterol, impede liver function, and in general exacerbate every cardiovascular risk factor imaginable. Also, these saturated fats tend to oxidize cells in the body, hence are suspected as a major cancer catalyst if consumed with excess relish and zest.

Polyunsaturated Fatty Acids (PUFAs)

The *poly* part comes from the fact that this type of fat has two or more double-bonded carbon molecules (omega-3 and omega-6) found in its structure, and thus two or more sites to support a hydrogen atom. Unsaturated PUFA fats are found only in plants, seeds, nuts, and the oils derived from them. I knew you were wondering.

PUFAs are plant oils, liquid at room temperature, that are derived primarily from such sources as almonds, borage, safflowers, non-GMO soybeans, sunflowers, walnuts, and other nuts and seeds, all of which contain the highest percentage of polyunsaturated fats found on the market today. These healthy fats help to lower bad cholesterol levels and act as blood thinners, thus reducing the risk of blood clots. PUFAs are also involved in the synthesis of countless valuable biochemical substances and agents critical to the task of emotional stability, internal organ functions, neurological relay, mental acuity (helpful in anxiety, depression, and prevention of Alzheimer's and Parkinson's diseases), and sensory perception. PUFAs fill you up, not out. PUFA foods help stabilize blood sugar; if consumed every two to three hours daily, they help keep insulin stable, hence help to burn excess body fat.

I always recommend at least 400 IUs of vitamin E daily to safeguard you from oxidation when you introduce PUFAs to your soon-to-be-long-lived, healthy lean-thigh life.

Monounsaturated Fats

Monounsaturated fat has one double-bonded carbon molecule in its structure, and thus one site to support a hydrogen atom. It is also an oil at room temperature and is derived from plant sources, such as avocadoes, olives, peanuts, and sesame seeds, as well as from some fish. It has all the properties and functions of polyunsaturated fat but is considered better at doing what it does. It's the most stable type of dietary fat to go for, and as a more stable fat, it will not oxidize as rapidly as a PUFA fat. Hence, monounsaturated fats are better for cooking and heating. Both PUFAs and monofats should be teamed together to reduce fat stores and burn, baby, burn!

Hydrogenated Fats

Aside from saturated fats, there are some other greasers you should have minimal-to-no contact with.

- Hydrogenated and partially hydrogenated fats. These are manmade, manufactured, unsaturated fats, such as margarine, that have been forced to take on more hydrogen atoms, thus activating cellular aging and becoming more devastating to your health.

- Heat-processed, refined fats and oils. These fats have little if any nutritional value and are quick to become rancid. First cold-pressed, unrefined, unprocessed fats and oils are excellent alternatives.

- Frying oils. These fats are used primarily with fast foods. They generally contain nasty chemical solvents that allow the oil to be used repeatedly at exorbitantly high temperatures for weeks and months on end.

- Trans fats. These are the worst kinds of hydrogenated oxidizing fats—repulsive, clog-your-heart killers. Avoid at all cost.

A word to the wise about margarine and most butter substitutes: Naturally occurring fatty acids have what is known as a cis configuration. Cis is a Latin prefix meaning on the same side. Trans is also a Latin prefix, which means on the other side. In order for a cis fatty acid to become a trans-fatty acid, it has to go to the other side, which is achieved via a manufacturing manipulation involving the addition of hydrogen atoms (hydrogenation). To make margarine, different oils are blended and altered to become a spreadable solid. This alteration occurs by using platinum and aluminum as catalysts to chemically add hydrogen to the blended oils, thus dragging them to the other side (think Darth Vader).

Consequently, not only is margarine a no-no nasty trans-fatty-acid Frankenstein creation, it is also generally contaminated with aluminum, one of the usual suspects for Alzheimer's disease (another reason you can believe it's not butter). Avoid hydrogenated and partially hydrogenated anything, as studies have shown they can lower your good HDL fats (not a good thing) and can increase your bad LDL fats.

Fat in Your Diet

Now you want to know how much fat to eat, right? Well, the average American woman currently gets about 37 percent of her calories from problem promoters such as saturated and hydrogenated fat. That's definitely too much of the bad fats for your butt and thighs. Bring your saturated-fat intake down and your unsaturated, monounsaturated, and PUFA healthy fat intake up to approximately 50 percent of your total calories daily and life will be groovy. Less than 5 percent should come from saturated fat. Again, the balance should be from thinning-for-your-thighs polyunsaturated combined with the good monounsaturated fat varieties.

For the average woman, if you use the caloric formulation value of 1,716 (weight of 143 pounds × 12 hours in a day = the number of calories needed), then approximately 50 percent, or 850 calories, should come from healthy essential omega-3, omega-6, and omega-9 fatty-acid foods and oils. That translates into approximately 90-plus grams of trim-down-your-bottom and thigh-firming EFAs per day. OK, enough calculations. Time to formulate a nutrient ratio. I recommend your daily caloric intake be divided this way:

- 30 percent lean bioavailable proteins

- 50 percent healthy EFA fats

- 20 percent low-glycemic carbohydrates (one-third from fruits, one-third from vegetables, and one-third from healthy, starchy carbohydrates)

I know, I know, you can't eyeball a percentage amount of calories either. Solution: When you eat, always make sure that at least 50 percent of the total calories going into your mouth during one meal are from the healthy EFAs. Your starchy carbohydrate portion should be the size of a kiwi or apple. And finally, your protein should be approximately the size of a deck of cards if consuming 1,200–1,400 calories daily. Or the size of two and a quarter decks of cards if on 1,800 calories. (*See* Appendix G for Daily Food Logs.)

VITAMINS AND MINERALS

When it comes to vitamins and minerals, the only issue I see involves whether or not you should take supplements. To that end, I have but one question to ask: Where have all the worms gone?

When I was a little girl, worms were everywhere. You couldn't walk down a sidewalk without seeing a big, fat banded one squirming and slithering around or getting pecked at by a robin. You couldn't go to school without some snot-nosed, boy creature trying to drop one down your blouse. What does this have to do with vitamins and minerals? Topsoil. Yep, it's all about dirt.

Topsoil, my lovelies, is the most agriculturally productive soil layer on the planet. It's what crops are grown in. Whatever is or isn't in the topsoil is or isn't in food. That's a simple correlation, right?

Every year in America, 1.8 billion tons of topsoil are lost from croplands. That's a government-supplied and verified statistic. See for yourself at www.soils.usda.gov/sqi/concepts/som.html. Some 120 million acres of farmland are eroding at a rate that exceeds the government's own established limits.

Worms live in topsoil. You don't see them anymore because the topsoil is lost or contaminated. Worms, as disgusting as you might find them, are crucial to the nutrient composition of soil. As it turns out, they're terrific composting critters, gobbling up organic matter and converting it into nourishing nutrients that the soil needs to grow foods high in nutrients.

Their castings (excreta) and tea (urine)—I'd stick with chamomile—are loaded with microorganisms that break down bacteria, fungus, and all sorts of other dirt matter into good, necessary vital nutrients. Their vermi-compost, as it's called, is rich in calcium, iron, manganese, magnesium, phosphorous, potassium, sodium, zinc, and most important, nitrogen. This is the most abundant gas in the atmosphere, making up 79 percent of the air floating around us (and you thought it was oxygen). Nitrogen is in every living plant or animal tissue because nothing, absolutely nothing, grows without nitrogen. Fertilizers are primarily designed to enhance the nitrogen content of the soil.

What worms do in topsoil affects the nutritional integrity of the entire food chain. So, the next time you see a worm, look at it, appreciate it, and don't step on it.

Did you know that, if you add enough nitrogen and water, you can grow a perfectly beautiful looking fruit or vegetable with just one seed, but—and here's the big but—it can be completely devoid of vitamins and minerals. Think organic. After learning about worms and soil erosion, you have to be questioning your food sources a bit. If you think what you're eating has all the nutrients you need to be a healthy lass, then I've got some real estate in Baghdad I'd like to sell you.

Remember this as well. The recommended daily allowances (the RDAs, or ridiculous daily allowances, as they're often referred to) sponsored by the USDA and the American Dietetic Association don't begin to insure that people consume even close to the amount of supplemental nutrients they really need.

The USDA (yep, the pyramid people) came up with RDAs in the 1940s by assessing the typical diets of twenty-three-year-old white American males who ate three squares a day. What about thirty-five-year-old Hispanic women, or sixty-year-old African-American men? Didn't they count, too?

Time has moved on. Things have changed. In fact, in 1992, the USDA

decided to change the RDA levels. It lowered them (hence the term ridiculous), despite the fact that almost 2 billion tons of topsoil are being lost every
year and the fact that twenty-three-year-old white males are a minority in
today's society. Enough said.

If you've got vitamin, mineral, and enzyme supplements, take them. Let
me worry about the yippity-yap coming from the nutrition naysayers out
there braying about having expensive urine due to the excretion of unutilized
vitamins and minerals. Do you want to know what the priciest pee really is?
It's the kind laced with all the overpriced prescription drugs people are wolf-
ing down.

Case in point: 45 percent of Americans take prescription drugs on a regular basis. As a result, trace elements of all kinds from pharmaceutical byproducts are winding up in municipal water supplies. You're drinking these
byproducts. They cannot be extracted by the less than up-to-date filtration
systems found in 90 percent of our cities and municipalities. Mexico isn't the
only country with straight-from-the-tap revenge.

This is one of the main reasons why your daughters are sprouting breasts
at ages seven or eight, and starting their menses far earlier than you did.
Think of all the estrogen and progesterone from all of those birth control
pills and hormone supplements that women have been ingesting and peeing
into the water supply for decades. And it doesn't seem likely that water-filtra-
tion plants will figure out how to remove these nasty byproducts anytime
soon, which is one very good reason to drink filtered, purified, reverse osmosis, or spring water whenever possible.

So, expensive-urine critics be damned. Besides, I'd rather have a glass of
water laced with trace elements of vitamin C and calcium over one laced with
pesticides and the metabolites from anti-depressants, diabetes drugs, or heart
medications any day.

You Can't Take It with You (And the Lies We've Been Told)

*F*at, in some respects, is like money. You need it, you want it, you save it, you spend it. And like Puff Daddy, P'Diddy, Diddy, or whatever he calls himself, and the notorious B.I.G. once said, *Mo money, mo problems.*

One thing is different, though. You can't leave your fat behind when you head for the Great Beyond. Unlike money, you can't bequeath blubber. Nobody in recorded history has ever left a sister or niece a saddlebag of jelly belly in a will. Besides, who would want it, anyway?

When you die (hopefully not for a long time), you won't need calories. It's not like you're going to spring up out of your coffin and run laps around the mausoleum or anything, so what good is your fat?

My advice: Use it while you can. Spend every chocolate-covered, crème-filled, mayonnaise, melted-butter, peach-cobbler, pecan-pie, and praline calorie you've got before you're gone because you can't take it with you. Time to burn what you've earned.

Speaking of burn, fat is a fuel. You know that. Fuel must be burned to be utilized. You know that, too. Oxygen helps fuel burn or expend through a process called combustion, which converts said fuel into heat and light (we're talking fifth grade science now). And how do we expose fat to oxygen so it can expend into heat and light? That's right, exercise. Move it or store it. You're probably glowing just thinking about this.

AEROBIC EXERCISE

What kind of exercise will allow for this much-desired combustion to take place? Aerobic exercise will, because aerobic means living or occurring in the presence of oxygen. Therefore, an aerobic exercise is any low-stress activity that requires an increased and sustained oxygen intake for steady fuel conversion and energy expenditure.

Got that? You have to do something to create a greater demand for oxygen, and you have to do it long enough for fat to be converted and expended as energy. How long, you ask? That's the best question yet.

Recall the whole short-term, long-term fuel explanation? (*See* Chapter 3.) Remember how I told you that glucose (short-term) gets used up first before fat (long-term)? And finally, remember how I told you that certain kinds of fat take a little bit more effort on the part of the body to be available for use, which is why they get stored more efficiently? Well, when doing aerobic exercise, your body initially operates on glucose. Depending on the amount of carbohydrate sugars consumed, it takes approximately thirty to forty minutes of aerobic cardiovascular exercise to move out of glucose burn. If the exercise is sustained long enough (fifty to seventy-five minutes) your body will begin to use stored fat for burning in anticipation of your glucose supply being exhausted. It takes twenty-six to thirty-five minutes for your fat-burning switch to turn on.

If you continue exercising beyond this switchover point, you will enter the fat zone. Here, you will burn fat exclusively as a fuel source. In other words, at the switchover point, you are at zero, and begin counting minutes for burning fat. This does not mean that shorter exercise periods will not assist your effort to reduce fat. All exercise helps. What it does mean is

How Fat Goes On and Off

Did you know that your body puts on and takes off fat in reverse order? No kidding. You put it on from toe to head and take it off from head to toe. That's why, when you start to gain, your britches get snug, and when you start to lose, your face gets more chiseled. Let your beautiful face lead the way.

that effective fat utilization occurs after glucose exhaustion. Train in the fat zone and your life will never be the same.

If you really want to tap into your fat (touch it, I'm sure you do), sustain any activity you can beyond twenty-six to twenty-eight minutes at 45 to 50 percent of your maximum heart rate (the aerobic-anaerobic threshold), called your target heart rate. Don't go crazy. Work up to this over a three-to-four-week cycle. The target heart rate is a metabolic trigger for the body to liberate fat as usable energy (free the fat, free the fat). It is also a level of cardiovascular activity that can be sustained for a protracted period. It's just high enough to get you heated and into sweat mode, but low enough to allow you to make like the Energizer bunny and just keep going and going and going. Remember, if you don't sweat, you're probably not hydrating or eating enough.

Now, before you begin fat-zone training, you must calculate your target heart rate. To do this, you simply need to subtract your age from 220 and take 50 and 60 percent of that number. The equations look like this:

(220 − age in years) × .50 = Low range of target heart rate
(220 − age in years) × .60 = High range of target heart rate

For the average American woman of 37, this means: 220 - 37 = 183. So, 50 to 60 percent of her maximum heart rate means a fat-zone target heart rate of 91–109 beats per minute.

The average American woman should strive to perform an exercise that will elevate her heart to this rate and sustain it beyond the twenty-six to twenty-eight minute switchover. She should also periodically check her heart rate while exercising, by using a monitoring device or by pressing her fingers to her wrist or carotid artery (either side of the neck near the voice box and counting the number of pulse beats in one minute.

Let me give you an example of how beautifully efficient fat-zone training is. Let's say, for example, that you ride a stationary bike for thirty minutes, five days a week, which means that each training day you are spending two to four minutes in the fat zone. By the end of the week, that represents a total of ten to twenty minutes of pure fat-burning.

Now, instead of thirty minutes, five days a week, attempt forty-five minutes for three days a week, which means that each training day you are spending seventeen to nineteen minutes in the fat zone. By the end of the week, that represents fifty-one to fifty-seven minutes of pure fat-burning—a three- to five-fold increase in actual fat expenditure. What if you trained four to five days a week for forty-five minutes, or fifty minutes, or an hour? Melt away, melt away, melt away all.

I don't mean to burst your bubble, but you've probably already heard that you have to burn off 3,500 calories to get rid of a pound of fat. Earlier I calculated that there were 4,086 calories in a pound of fat (that 3,500 looks a bit more appealing doesn't it?). Aha, lest you forget, fat is about 13 percent water. So, it is true that 454 grams equals one pound of fat. But by subtracting the water percentage, you get a truer fat yield of 395 grams, or 3,555 calories. Close enough. So what is the very best exercise for fat zone training? Walking is.

Walking

You can do it anywhere, it doesn't cost anything but time, it accommodates a broad fitness range, it allows for easy heart-rate monitoring and, like the aforementioned Energizer Bunny, when you walk, you can keep going and going and going.

Walking is best when focused on time and not necessarily distance. The longer you go at your target heart rate, the more fat you will burn. Also, try a yogic style of walking called breath walk, which involves breathing at a prescribed rate and at prescribed intervals. Check out www.cyberjaz.com/szabo/breath.htm for more about breathing exercises. The rate at which you breathe is also a metabolic trigger for what kind of fuel your body elects to use.

ANAEROBIC EXERCISE

There is another type of exercise you can do that will dramatically assist your fat-reduction efforts, and help you stay lean forever. It's anaerobic exercise.

I can hear you thinking, *Isn't that the opposite of aerobic exercise?* Yes, it is. Anaerobic means living or occurring in the absence of oxygen. Therefore, an anaerobic exercise is any high-stress activity, such as weightlifting, that does not require an increased and sustained oxygen intake for sudden fuel conver-

Incredible Fat Trivia for Walking

Fat is partly water. As it burns, the water part of it is liberated into the bloodstream, which means you're eventually going to excrete it. The water that comes by way of ingestion serves the purpose of hydration. So, if you drink while you're walking, you'll actually use that water to prevent dehydration. The water being liberated from fat goes to the bladder. So, move until you have to *go*, that way you'll really know you burned fat. Stride until your bladder is full. And when you *go*, you'll be amazed at how clear your urine is. It's fat water. Also, the more fat you lose, the longer it will take for your bladder to fill up when you exercise, a sign that you're getting leaner.

sion and energy expenditure. You're wondering how this can help when you need to burn long-term fuel. Such an inquisitive mind you have. Just keep those questions coming.

Let me break it down nice and easy for you. Your lean tissue—bones, internal organs, muscles, and skin—is active tissue. This means your body makes a great effort to build, nourish, clean, repair, and maintain it, an effort collectively referred to as metabolic activity or metabolism. Fat, on the other hand, is an inactive substance (lazy, greasy, yellow stuff) and does not require much effort by your body to sustain.

Your metabolic activity utilizes energy, which, for the body, is measured in calories. The more lean or active tissue in your body, the more metabolic activity that occurs to sustain it, and consequently, the more calories you will utilize. This is most desirable if you do not wish to be a fat-body person.

One pound of muscle requires about 30 calories a day to be sustained, whereas one pound of fat only needs 3 to 5. What this means is that the more muscle you have, the higher your BMR (basil metabolic rate)—you literally burn more calories throughout the day than a high-body-fat individual. What this also means is that the more muscle you have, the more you can eat before gaining weight or putting on fat. Yeah, baby. Kind of makes you want to go pump some iron, doesn't it?

Anaerobic exercise, characterized by brief high-stress activity, helps to increase your body's lean tissue mass. The term high-stress does not mean negative and harmful activity. It refers to adaptive stress or the type of stress that stimulates your body to adjust to greater demands. One way to adjust is by building more lean tissue (hypertrophy).

Weight Training

The most common form of anaerobic exercise is weight training, which falls under the more general category of progressive resistance training. The stress registered by the effort to overcome a weight or other resistance forces your body to adapt by building more muscle and bone (think avoid osteoporosis) to assist the effort. As you adapt and go on to increase the weight or resistance (hence, progressive resistance), the effort will spur on the development of more lean tissue. This is A + B = C stuff.

Weight training does not equate with bodybuilding, a sport characterized by a dramatic (some say freakish) alteration in muscular appearance. Just because you pick up a dumbbell doesn't mean you will be transformed into a world-class muscle-head. You control the dumbbell just like you wield the fork. Either way, you ultimately control how you look.

However, weight training, Pilates, and certain types of yoga are methods of body sculpting or shaping that can be great nonsurgical approaches to creating a more desirable you. And for those of you who might be afraid of lifting a little weight, you should be aware that a pound of fat can take up five times more space than a pound of muscle. Ask yourself this question: *Do I have five times more butt than I need?* I'll see you in the gym.

GLUCOSE DEPLETION

If you've never heard of glucose depletion, you're not alone. Most people are not familiar with this concept. Basically, it means manipulating your food intake relative to exercise, in order to teach your body to burn, rather than store, fat. Can this really be done? I'll answer that question with a question. Do you believe anybody really can become president? Of course it can be done.

You know that exhausting the glucose available in your bloodstream will force your body to tap into its fat reserves. Well, glucose depletion takes this physiological cause-and-effect and uses it as an exercise strategy to train your body to utilize rather than store fat—even when you're not exercising.

Quite simply, the day before you do fat-zone aerobic work, greatly restrict, if not completely eliminate, your intake of high-glycemic, starchy carbohydrates. This will create a glucose debt, which will force your body to be more determined about accessing its fat reserves upon exercising.

The reverse of this, glucose storing, is what endurance athletes (marathon runners, triathletes) engage in prior to competition. The day before an event, they do carbohydrate loading (they pig-out on pasta, potatoes, and rice) to insure they will have an abundance of easy-access glucose/glycogen to fuel them. This is a critical concern since these athletes have very low body-fat reserves, hence faster metabolisms.

The fat-utilization effectiveness of glucose depletion has long been recognized by bodybuilders, fitness stars, and many a body-conscious celebrity. This type of training will convert your body from one that stores fat to one that burns it, constantly—and this is a good thing.

NITROGEN BALANCE

Let me get you up to speed on what nitrogen balance is all about. And no, this has nothing to do with trying to steady a molecule on the tip of your finger.

Quick definition: Nitrogen is an odorless, colorless gas that makes up about 79 percent of our atmosphere; nothing grows without it, and it can be found in the tissues of all living things.

So, you're asking yourself, *What does nitrogen have to do with me and my fat?* Fortunately for you, I know the answer and I'm willing to share it. You can thank me later.

If your body retains more nitrogen than it excretes, it will establish a positive nitrogen balance. This will accelerate the building process for lean tissue, just like fertilizers do for plants by creating a positive nitrogen balance in soil.

But, you ask, *What if I'm not interested in increasing my lean tissue? What if I just want to get rid of my fat and keep my lean tissue as it is? What about nitrogen then?* I'm quite impressed by these shrewd questions, but you still need to be concerned about creating and sustaining a positive-nitrogen balance, just to preserve the lean tissue you have.

This is especially of concern when doing aerobic training. While aerobic exercise is good for fat reduction, it is bad for preserving your muscles. You see, muscle, like everything else, undergoes a chemical alteration when it is exposed to oxygen (when oxidation occurs). Rebellious chemicals, unpaired electrons known as free radicals, are created and begin attacking cell membranes, resulting in a breakdown of muscle tissue (catabolism). This is why meat weighs less and looks and tastes differently after being cooked (cooking is an oxidative process). In fact, many people who do a lot of aerobic training lose skin and muscle tone and look aged because their tissue is being heavily oxidized by the increased oxygen intake. Now you know why you have never seen a 280-pound, muscle-bound marathon runner.

This is also why supplements called antioxidants are highly promoted as nutritional aids. If you can retard or prevent the side effects of oxidation, you will age more slowly and preserve the composition of your tissue. You want this, and a positive nitrogen balance is what creates this desirable counter-effect. The key to this creation is so easy, you won't believe it—eat more greens. Yup, it's that simple. Organic green beet tops, chard, collards, kale, spinach, and other green vegetables that come right out of the rich soil are loaded with nitrogen. Another way to elevate your nitrogen count is to increase your intake of lean bioavailable proteins, because protein is rich in nitrogen. Still another simple way to create a positive nitrogen balance is to eat gelatin. It is pure protein. This is why it helps to grow nails and hair.

How will you know if you have achieved a positive nitrogen balance? Well, other than the visible reality of a leaner, more youthful appearance, you won't know unless you check for it via a urine sample. This can be done by a physician (unnecessary expense) or by purchasing nitrogen strips (chemically sensitive paper that changes color to indicate nitrogen amounts) and testing yourself. You can buy them at health food stores. Now you don't have to worry about breaking down your muscle tissue (catabolizing yourself).

When you embark on this comprehensive fat-reduction effort that includes eating, healthy lifestyle shifts, and exercise, I don't recommend dropping more than ten pounds at a time. Set your mind on an amount greater than that and you'll end up falling for those starvation sucker diets. I've already explained what will happen if you do that. You're too smart for that old ploy. Your mama didn't raise a fool.

A slower, more gradual reduction of fat creates less shock to your system, which keeps the metabolic finger off the fat-storage button. It also allows for your body to adjust to the alteration without interpreting it as a survival threat. Besides, what's the rush? Everyone's been duped into thinking that quick weight loss is a good thing. It's about as good as quick blood loss, which is favorably viewed only by leeches, mosquitoes, and vampires.

Look at it this way. If you put on twenty-five pounds of rump over the last five years, but took steps to burn off a pound of fat a week, all that extra butt would be gone in half a year. That's one-tenth the time it took you to put it on, and that's pretty good in my book.

Focus on burning off one to two pounds of fat a week. You'll get there. The key is consistency. If you roll off the wagon, hop back on the next day. Self-chastisement is a waste of good energy that would be best put into a brisk stroll of twenty to thirty minutes.

FYI: Exercise can also help your body combat stress, and this can keep you from porking up. Pressure, worry, and anxiety stimulate the production of stress chemicals such as adrenaline and cortisol, which activate our flight-or-fight survival response, hence promoting the storing of more fat. (*See* Appendix E for additional information on cortisol.)

You see, back in our Paleolithic glory days, long before we had running shoes, attorneys, and pepper spray, we had to either run from a threat or fight it. Both involve movement. Stress chemicals, particularly cortisol, stimulate your nervous system, muscles, and heart and also elevate your blood sugar levels to enable that movement. If elevated chemicals and no movement, then bingo—stored fat. An elevated blood-sugar level isn't all that it's cracked up to be.

If you move, as in exercise, you use these stress chemicals. This is one of the reasons you feel more at ease after a jog on the lakefront. If you don't move, you won't release and use the chemicals, and they will continuously send a signal to your body to do something, which is why your muscles tighten when you're anxious.

These chemicals will also continuously signal a demand for more blood sugar, which gets the insulin going, which again causes more fat storage, especially in the omentum. Remember, eat the apple, don't become one. As long as you exercise, you won't have to worry about this. Worry—get it?

The Absolute Absolute

I would like to share something with you at this moment. Believe it or not, I was once a French-fry fiend, a sour-cream-stuffing, sauce-and-syrup-smothering, Snickers-bar, saturated-fat sinner myself. In the past, I frequented many calorie houses of ill repute: the greasy spoons, the doughnut shops, the all-you-can-eat diners and the beer gardens of iniquity. I'm not proud of this. But I have to be honest with you, and I'm asking you to be honest with yourself.

My past indiscretions provided me with hard lessons that have led me to my current life of dietary redemption, and I now have the knowledge, the power, and the will to prevail. In all my years, I have come to learn there is one concrete, irrefutable, undeniable, absolute truth about weight control, and it trumps all the knowledge, in all the books, in all the world that you could ever read.

I'm ready to share it with you, but only if you really want to do away with those Häagen-Dazhooligans that inhabit your hips; only if you are truly honest about your desire to walk away from the corpulent corruption that has checkered your past; and only if you are passionate about purging your mind of the potato-chip perversions that have compromised every *I'm going to do it this time* promise you have ever made to yourself. If you are willing to swear to adhere to the one tenet that is paramount to all others, with all the cross-your-heart, miracle-bra commitment you can muster, then girlfriend, I'm ready to give it you.

Never, ever, ever, ever, ever buy bigger clothes. If you buy bigger clothes, you will fill them up.

This is the single greatest piece of advice I have to offer regarding weight control. Unless you are gestating and your burgeoning body dimensions are bringing new life into the world, don't do it.

Some women have four different dress sizes in their closets right now. But all the nutritional knowledge and exercise information I could ever give you will be as meaningless as serving you a large plate of fries with a Twinkie side if you buy bigger clothes. That's real. That's the truth and Sister-Self will back me up on this.

There you have it—a hundred-plus pages, just as I said. I kept my word. Now it's your turn to keep yours. My hope is that you don't dig your grave with a spoon. Do what you know you need to do to bring the best *you* forward. I believe you can and I have a strong, good, gut feeling you will.

And always remember: The only thing you want to fatten up is your bank account.

Still not convinced? Read on.

Case Histories with Successful Outcomes

*T*he folks in this chapter "looked in the mirror," took charge of themselves, and learned how to "eat, sleep, and excrete" properly. Use the knowledge and tools that follow and you *can* be the abundantly healthy, happy, lean person you want to be—when you take charge of *you.*

STUBBORN FAT MELTS WITH DIETARY TRIAGE

Frances, a thirty-three-year-old mother of a twenty-one-month-old boy, sought nutrition therapy with the goals of losing fifty pounds of pregnancy weight and improving her severe lack of energy. She complained of constipation, chronic pain, excessive urination, frequent dizziness, painful intercourse, and pesky PMS symptoms involving extreme moodiness and cravings for lots of chocolate (otherwise her life was perfect).

Her diet was packed with coffee, sugar, and daily chocolate treats. Seventy-three percent of her food choices of less than optimal sustenance consisted of 73 percent carbohydrates—way too high. These high-sugar, low-fiber, fat-storing carbohydrates, such as cookies, goldfish crackers, pasta, and white rice, were her doom. She averaged a 12-percent intake of proteins, far too low for a breastfeeding mama. Her healthy fatty-acid intake was 0 percent, while her saturated-fat intake rolled in at 14 percent of her total daily intake. Healthy fats were not even a concept. Her daily intake of fiber, 6–7 grams, was woefully under the ideal of 30-plus grams per day—small wonder that she moved toward the more constipated side of the fence. Her water intake was a measly six cups a day, while she needed a minimum of twelve cups daily to even begin bolstering her metabolism and lose weight.

We shifted Frances's caloric intake to 30 percent proteins, 50 percent essential fatty acids, and 20 percent high-fiber, low-glycemic carbohydrates; we cut out the coffee and set scheduled treat times in an attempt to satisfy her need for a rendezvous with her sweet treat of choice. Our goal was to have her sinfully nosh one or two times a week at most, whether on a cookie, a chunk o' chocolate, or a latte.

After five months on this regime, Frances's body fat had melted from 35 to 22 percent, while her weight had dropped from 165 to 125 and she had lost 32.7 pounds of fat. On a scale of 1–10, her energy zoomed from 3 to 10, primarily due to diet shifts and going to bed by 10 P.M. instead of 2 A.M. Lights out and early to bed helps lower cortisol levels and stabilize the hormone insulin, which in turn encourages consistent fat burning.

Frances, who continues her beneficial routine to this day, now looks like her saucy pre-pregnancy self and has created incredible energy to keep up with her very active toddler.

COOKING CLASS CHANGES EVERYTHING FOR THE BETTER

Natasha, a darling thirty-five-year-old mom of three very active boys under the age of six, ran her husband's growing, and very demanding, real estate development company out of their hectic home. On a 0–10 scale, her overall energy was a measly 4, with 10 as the ideal. She lived on coffee, consumed little-to-no water, experienced migraines at least twice a week, had little-to-no sex drive, and feared her monthly cycle, which was always accompanied by cramping, excessive bleeding, bruising, and scary moodiness and depression. At 5 feet tall, she felt her weight should have been 105–110 pounds instead of 120 pounds. Her body fat was 33.5 percent, which meant she carried 40.2 pounds of fat on her petite frame. She was doing Pilates once a week and eating maybe 400–600 calories a day. (With too much exercise and not enough food who wouldn't have migraines?)

When Natasha came to me, her goals were to increase her energy and sex drive, plus lose her excess fat, as well as the crippling migraines. Time was a total commodity for her so we did a grocery store walkabout to introduce her to quick, throw-together options for her and the kids in an attempt to create more ease in her daily living. She then took the How to Cook for a Week in Less than One Hour Cooking Class that I offer. It changed her life.

Within five months of eating a minimum of 1,200–1,300 calories a day, her energy had shot up and was consistently a 10. Her weight was down to 110 and her body fat was down to 24 percent, bringing her total pounds of fat to 26.4 pounds versus her previous 40.2 pounds. She had lost 13.8 pounds of fat and had increased her lean mass by 3.8 pounds.

After the third month, her period was a nonissue, and best of all, she had no more migraines. Her husband even called to personally thank me for giving him back his beautiful, sexy wife who once again thought he was the best thing next to her time-saving washer and dryer.

To support her nonstop, fourteen-hour days, I gradually increased her to 1,500–1,600 calories a day, and up to this moment, she is still lean and still running full-steam-ahead, with a healthy libido to boot!

BACK FROM THE BRINK

Dennis, a forty-year-old father of four, had big concerns regarding his health. He had put on thirty-one pounds over five years and was inspired to seek nutrition therapy as two of his closest friends in their forties and fifties had recently died.

He had aches and pains, allergies, high blood pressure, low energy, and 42.9 percent body fat (under 18 percent is ideal for men). He worked long days, ate late, and slept short nights, retiring about midnight or 1 A.M., the combination of which can increase body fat and arterial plaque exponentially while simultaneously creating efficient fat storage.

He ate only two meals a day, but they consisted of salty fast and convenient foods on the go. The six to eight cups of water he drank daily were buttressed by half a gallon of Diet Coke (talk about bloat and excess water weight). His diet was 50 percent protein, 30 percent saturated fat, and 47 percent high-sugar carbohydrates, with zero intake of healthy essential fatty acids (EFAs).

We actually increased his total calories, but made sure they were comprised of more optimal proportions than before—50 percent EFAs, 30 percent protein, and 20 percent high-fiber, low-glycemic carbohydrates. His water intake was increased to one gallon a day and in two weeks he was off the diet soda. He started out walking twenty minutes a day and gradually increased that to two hours daily. Instead of going to bed late, he started eating earlier, getting to sleep by 10:30 P.M., and averaging eight hours of sleep.

After just two months on this regimen, Dennis's weight had dropped from 281 to 264 pounds, his body fat was down from 42 to 31 percent (118 pounds of fat to 81.3 pounds), and his lean mass went up from 163 pounds to 182.1 pounds. His blood pressure went down into the normal range, his aches and pains were greatly reduced, the shortness of breath disappeared, and he regained his energy.

His family was so thrilled about his improved health that they joined him in his healthy diet and exercise routine, and they are all now experiencing results similar to his in terms of weight loss and energy.

BALANCED EATING PROGRAM TO THE RESCUE

Suzie was a fifty-two-year-old woman who, although physically active and practicing what she thought was pretty good nutrition, was very overweight. In her early forties, she had begun to experience the beginnings of several health challenges, including a carcinoma of the left breast. Then came osteopenia. At forty-seven, she noticed her hips had became very stiff and inflexible. Five years later, a periodic irregular heartbeat was discovered during an examination after she had fainted. That's when she knew she needed to do something different. She scheduled a nutrition consultation with me to take off her thirty extra pounds, bolster her immunity, and rid herself of her unending stiffness.

Under my tutelage, Suzie learned to eat more nutritious and balanced meals—bolstered by three snacks a day—that exponentially improved her health on all levels. Her energy level increased 100 percent, her heartbeat maintained regularity, and the flexibility and strength in her hips were significantly improved. In addition, and most relevant to this book, in the course of five months, Suzie dropped thirty-four pounds. She now glowingly reports that by diligently following my eating program (30 percent proteins/50 percent fats/20 percent carbohydrates)—especially by consuming the necessary amounts of essential fatty acids in foods and oils—while continuing her workouts (aerobics, Pilates, strength training, and yoga), her quality of life has improved by leaps and bounds.

CAREFUL REGIMEN RESTORES FORMER LUSTER

Andrea, a sixty-nine-year-old woman, was 5'2" and weighed in at 192 pounds of evenly distributed weight when she arrived for a consultation. An Italian Sophia-Loren type, with huge doe eyes and eyelashes that looked too heavy to hold up, you could see she had been considered beautiful all her life. Besides having far too many pounds on her once-lithe frame, her biggest issues were a hiatal hernia, chronic bronchitis, bad diarrhea, rheumatoid arthritis, bad psoriasis on her hands, and bunions and nerve damage in both her feet. Phew— she had some issues.

Andrea's diet consisted mostly of chocolate. Chocolate for breakfast, lunch, dinner, and a snack or two. Obviously addicted to chocolate, she was powerless over her addiction. Poor thing. Her calories were ample but empty, offering no-to-low nutritional support. Although she said she loved to eat and loved to cook, she lived alone so found it easier to grab chocolate than cook for one.

I set her up to do the following: practice only water-based exercise for the first two to three weeks; begin using products to reduce inflammation of the feet, hands, and intestines; get off chocolate altogether within two weeks; begin acupuncture; shift food choices to live, eaten-as-they-are-grown foods; take digestive anti-inflammatory enzyme support, six tabs three times a day, exactly ten minutes before each meal; and consume lots of fiber. To further decrease inflammation, 60 percent of her daily calories were to come from healthy fats and oils.

Andrea's goal was to lighten her load and in six months go off to Italy to see an old flame. I felt she could easily drop six pounds a month, even without consistent exercise. Her body fat was 45.3 percent, while the total number of pounds of fat rolled in at 89.6. The goal she and I set together was to lose 35 to 40 pounds in six months. We had some work to do.

By the fourth month, Andrea had dropped from 198 to 166 pounds and she quickly got up to thirty minutes of walking a day, while having physical therapy three times a week. She broke a sweat every day and increased her water intake from two to twelve cups daily. By six months, Andrea had reduced her body fat from 45.3 percent to 32 percent, and had a total loss of 36.5 pounds of pure fat. The skin on her hands was as beautiful as the skin on her face, her stools were at least 20 inches daily, and her arthritis was provoked only when she nibbled on chocolate. By the time she was ready for her trip, she looked fifteen years younger. Look out Italy!

MOM TIMES TWO AFTER TURNAROUND

Kathy's stated goals when she came to me were to lose weight by reducing her body fat from 35 to 25 percent and to increase her energy, which at the time was a lowly 4 on a scale of 0–10. She really wanted to move her bowels more than three times a week and find the key to sleeping through the night.

She lived on Diet Coke, drank four to five grande lattes daily and consumed three to four alcoholic beverages three to five times a week, while eating around 1,000 calories in food per day. She had ongoing inflammation in her muscles and back (her biggest problem), and said if we could work on that, she would be most appreciative. Also, as she was thirty-six years old, she very much wanted to get pregnant within the next year. Her stress level was enormous, she said, and her workdays were long (thirteen hours plus), so she wanted to sell her business.

Sleep was my number-one priority for her since without it she would neither heal nor lose weight. Within two weeks, I had her sleeping like a baby eight to nine hours a night (her bedtime down to 10 P.M. versus her previous habit of turning in at midnight or 1 A.M.).

She weaned herself off Diet Coke and coffee, and chose to limit her alcohol intake to one or two times a week, with no more than one to two drinks each time. She increased her water intake, averaging ten to twelve cups a day, and eventually moved 18 inches of stool through her bowels every day. I gradually increased her total daily calories to 1,400, 50 percent of them from essential fatty acids, 30 percent from proteins, and 20 percent from high-fiber, low-glycemic carbohydrates. She also increased her exercise time from sporadic to a committed forty-five minutes three times a week. After all, she finally had energy.

By three weeks, all her back and muscle aches were completely gone. By four weeks, she had dropped to 125 pounds, while her body fat had melted down to 27 percent—she went from 47.2 to 33.7 pounds of fat.

Due to a prior diagnosis of polycystic ovaries, Kathy had been told it would not be easy for her to get pregnant. But she fooled them and is now on her second, healthy pregnancy. She loves being mostly at home as a semi-retired, non-caffeinated, H_2O-drinking, lean, energetic mom.

BEING GOOD TO HERSELF TOO

Marianna was a 5'2", fifty-six-year-old, 156-pound stay-at-home mom who still had a few of her grown-up flock living in the nest. Being the good mother, she continued to cook, clean, shop, launder, iron, and, in general, take care of everyone but herself. This created enormous stress levels that helped pack on the pounds. She was a chronic faster and dieter, so much so that she developed scurvy (primarily on her back) from a long-term vitamin-C deficiency.

Marianna's goal was to learn how to take care of herself, with healthy eating and exercise, and drop her body fat, a total of 56 pounds, from 36 percent to 26 percent. She was aiming for 130 pounds on the scale, and to achieve this, I recommended a forty-five minute walk five days a week, yoga to increase flexibility, and meditation and breath work for stress reduction. I also bumped her meager 600-calorie daily intake up to a minimum of 1,300–1,400 calories daily.

As her skin was absurdly dry, I started out having 65 percent of these calories come from foods high in EFAs, primarily avocados, hummus, and raw nuts and seeds, all of which have healing, fat-burning essential oils. After three weeks, when I lowered her EFA intake to 50 percent of her daily calories, her weight went down to 149 pounds and her body fat measured 30 percent. Thirteen weeks after shifting her awareness and finally eating enough, Marianna reached her goal of a lean, lovely physique. Plus, in her new-found determination to be good to herself too, she helped move two of her three chicks out of the nest.

Appendices

Your Tool Kit to Getting the Skinny on Fat

Appendix A

Information on Food

THE GOOD, THE BAD, AND THE UGLY
IN PROTEINS, FATS, AND CARBOHYDRATES

The three-dimensional Enlightened Food Pyramid is quite simply *sensible*!

They are the girlfriend's guide to awakening your consciousness to the Good, the Bad, and the Truly Ugly foods found abudantly everywhere in America.

These *ugly, seductive* taste-bud teasers are like crack cocaine. Once you nosh on these tempting titillating taste-teasers, your brain acts like a runaway train going faster and faster, heading for disaster.

The good-for-you, thigh-thinning, hormone-balancing, blood-sugar–stabilizing, cholesterol-lowering, immune-enhancing foods are located at the largest portion of each pyramid—the base.

- These foods are the *foundation* upon which to build your road to excellent long-term health.

- These foods are the *fix-what's-wrong-with-you* healthy proteins, fats, and carbohydrates.

Allow yourself a cheat date once a week—*not daily*—and you will zip to the head of the class in the game called life!

PROTEINS

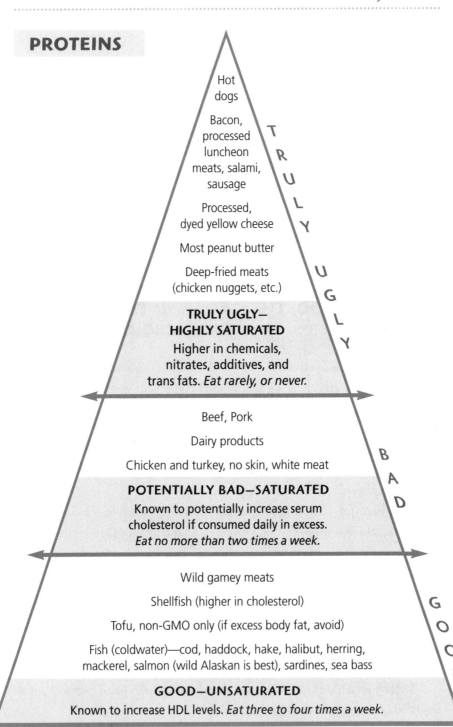

Hot dogs

Bacon, processed luncheon meats, salami, sausage

Processed, dyed yellow cheese

Most peanut butter

Deep-fried meats (chicken nuggets, etc.)

**TRULY UGLY—
HIGHLY SATURATED**
Higher in chemicals, nitrates, additives, and trans fats. *Eat rarely, or never.*

Beef, Pork

Dairy products

Chicken and turkey, no skin, white meat

POTENTIALLY BAD—SATURATED
Known to potentially increase serum cholesterol if consumed daily in excess. *Eat no more than two times a week.*

Wild gamey meats

Shellfish (higher in cholesterol)

Tofu, non-GMO only (if excess body fat, avoid)

Fish (coldwater)—cod, haddock, hake, halibut, herring, mackerel, salmon (wild Alaskan is best), sardines, sea bass

GOOD—UNSATURATED
Known to increase HDL levels. *Eat three to four times a week.*

T R U L Y *U G L Y*

B A D

G O O D

FATS

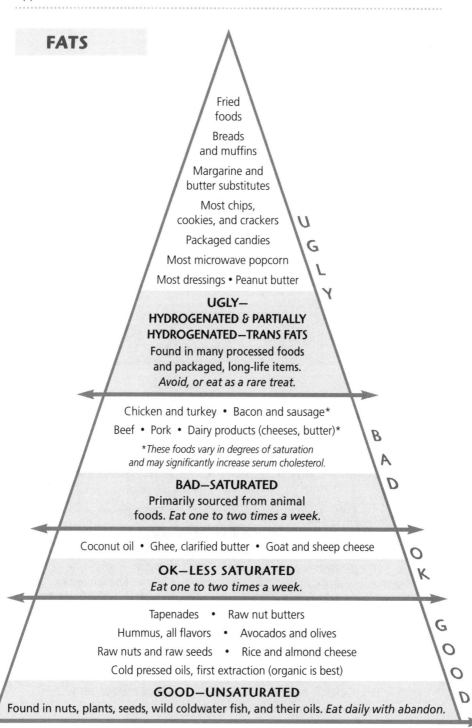

Fried
foods

Breads
and muffins

Margarine and
butter substitutes

Most chips,
cookies, and crackers

Packaged candies

Most microwave popcorn

Most dressings • Peanut butter

**UGLY—
HYDROGENATED & PARTIALLY
HYDROGENATED—TRANS FATS**
Found in many processed foods
and packaged, long-life items.
Avoid, or eat as a rare treat.

Chicken and turkey • Bacon and sausage*
Beef • Pork • Dairy products (cheeses, butter)*

*These foods vary in degrees of saturation
and may significantly increase serum cholesterol.*

BAD—SATURATED
Primarily sourced from animal
foods. *Eat one to two times a week.*

Coconut oil • Ghee, clarified butter • Goat and sheep cheese

OK—LESS SATURATED
Eat one to two times a week.

Tapenades   •   Raw nut butters
Hummus, all flavors   •   Avocados and olives
Raw nuts and raw seeds   •   Rice and almond cheese
Cold pressed oils, first extraction (organic is best)

GOOD—UNSATURATED
Found in nuts, plants, seeds, wild coldwater fish, and their oils. *Eat daily with abandon.*

U G L Y

B A D

O K

G O O D

CARBOHYDRATES

All
sodas,
regular
and diet,
alcohol, coffee

Wheat Thins,
Doritos, Fritos,
Snack products,
cookies, pretzels,
microwave popcorn,

Packaged juices
high in fructose (corn)
Corn-sweetened anything!

SUPER DOUGH BOY
Convert readily to fat—
many additives and chemicals.

T R U L Y   U G L Y

Most cereals, low fiber, high sugar
Pasta • Rice Cakes • Bagels and muffins
Anything white (bread, pasta, potato, rice, etc.)
Most breads, low fiber, high maltose (type of sugar)

THE UGLY–DOUGH BOY, THIGH PLUMPERS

U G L Y

Corn or popcorn (non-GMO, organic only)
Oats • Kavli crackers • Matzo crackers • Pitas • Tortillas

THE BAD–OK IN MODERATION
Eat one to two times a week. Wheat is the number two
ranking allergen, and 93 percent of the population is allergic to
gluten, the springy protein found in oats, rye, wheat, and white rice.

B A D

Garnet yams and squashes
Starchy vegetables (includes beets, carrots, peas, and sweet potatoes)
Vegetables and fruits • Legumes and beans • Rice crackers (not cakes)
Whole grains (includes amaranth, brown and wild rice, kamut, millet, quinoa)

THE GOOD–MUSCLE BUILDING–HIGH IN NUTRIENTS
Eaten as they are grown, moderate on glycemic index. *Eat daily.*

G O O D

BASIC RULES OF THE ROAD

1. **Drink enough water.** To calculate what you need per day:

   Weight in pounds × .075 = number of cups of water

2. **Know your body's protein requirements.** To calculate how many ounces of protein you require daily (the minimum number of grams of protein your body needs):

   Weight in pounds ÷ 2 = ounces of protein needed daily

   If you work out for one hour six to seven days a week, you should divide by 1.5 instead of 2:

   Weight in pounds ÷ 1.5 = ounces of protein needed daily

Note: There are 7 grams of protein in:

   ✔ 1 ounce of animal protein

   ✔ $1\frac{1}{2}$ ounce of coldwater fish

   ✔ 2 ounces low fat cottage cheese

   ✔ two egg whites

   ✔ one whole egg

   ✔ 3 ounces tofu
   Soy: Consume non-GMO (genetically modified products, organism-free) only! Be aware that soy is a top allergen. Consume rarely, not daily, and only if you are lean and/or postmenopausal.

---

3. **Consume essential edible oils in three divided doses at breakfast, lunch, and dinner.** Eating between 1.5 teaspoons and 1 tablespoon three times a day is ideal. *Do not count heated oils.* Always consume healthy EFAs with a protein-based meal for optimal utilization.

4. **Try to consume at least two to four pieces of fresh fruit, and 2–4 cups of steamed vegetables daily.** All foods mentioned above are low

on the glycemic index and high in fiber and water, all of which helps to burn fat, stabilize insulin, and build more lean mass.

5. **Eat enough total calories for your body's daily minimum requirements.** To calculate your daily caloric needs use this formula:

Weight in pounds $\times$ [active hours in your day] = number of calories needed per day

To lose one pound of fat per week, lower your calorie consumption, take the total found in the equation above, minus 500 calories. To lose one half to one more pounds per week, burn 250–500 more calories per day with exercise.

6. **If you can't obtain foods that are ideal, eat what is available; just be sensible.**

7. **Exercise.** If nothing else, walk at least three times a week. Start with fifteen to twenty minutes and work up to forty-five to sixty minutes.

8. **Attempt to eat an EFA food every two to three hours without fail.** This regulates insulin, hence burns fat, even if you are sedentary.

9. **Feel free to consume more healthy EFA foods at each feeding if you are still hungry.** High-fiber foods are the next best choice.

10. **If you miss one of your fatty acid snacks:** Try to load these fat units into the prior feeding, if possible, or load them into the meal following the snack. Always make up missed units/calories, whatever the category.

11. **Do not eat fewer units or calories than calculated.** You will not lose body fat readily, however you will lose precious muscle mass.

12. **You may always eat more.** Simply consume more healthy fats as a first choice, then select vegetables before you load up on carbohydrates and proteins.

13. **If you can't give up caffeinated products or if you intend to wean yourself off them:** Consume coffee or caffeine products three hours *after* your morning protein drink or a high healthy-fat breakfast—not *before*. *Never* on an empty stomach!

14. **Eat small feedings every two to three hours.** Preferably, you should eat an EFA or healthy-fat food. This keeps your insulin levels stable and helps burn stored fats.

ESSENTIAL FATTY ACIDS VERSUS NON-ESSENTIAL FATTY ACIDS

Essential fatty acids are essential because:

- Your body needs them to maintain health (for maintenance of immune function).

- Your body can't make them. They must come from the foods you eat.

- Eating patterns have changed radically over the last hundred years. Americans now face a subtle form of famine: The American diet has produced starvation of vital nutrients and a critical lack of healthy fats and essential amino acids for the body. Highly developed civilized cultures have supermarkets packed with boxes, freezers, and cans of anything and everything, yet upon consumption our bodies continue to be starved of vital nutrients, especially essential fatty acids (EFAs). Hence cravings.

  - EFAs are found in many foods, but they are most abundant in pure oils derived from certain nuts, seeds, legumes, and coldwater fish.

  - EFAs are fragile, easily damaged by air, high temperatures, and food processing. Most oil consumed today has been heavily processed or cooked/fried until it not only has few nutrients left but often oxidizes your precious cells on contact.

  - EFA need increases even more if you eat the wrong kind of fats and if you don't get enough of certain essential vitamins and minerals, the lack of which may render your body unable to make proper use of the EFAs you do consume.

  - EFAs come in two varieties: saturated and unsaturated. Most saturated fatty acids you consume are unnecessary. Not only do they clog up your arteries but consuming excess unhealthy saturated EFAs can interfere with your body's ability to use supportive healthy EFAs. (Saturated fats, such as beef fat and hard cheese, are stiff and hard at room temperature. Just imagine what these do to your arteries and heart.)

Not All Unsaturated Fatty Acids Are Essential

Watch out for hydrogenated products. The hydrogenation process, used to prolong shelf life, converts saturated fats into nasty unsaturated transfats. Avoid partially unsaturated (partially hydrogenated) products. They are actually worse, as the manufacturing process physically alters any EFAs in the oil, creating artificial trans-fatty acids mixed with saturated fats. These artificial fatty acids have far-reaching negative consequences on your health.

The Best Oils to Use in Cooking

When reaching for an oil to use for cooking with heat, choose from this list first:

- Coconut, ghee (clarified butter), olive, and sesame oils are the most stable, hence the best oils to use in cooking.

- For the best dressings use omega-3, omega-6, and omega-9 organic oil blends: safflower, sunflower (high in omega-6 EFAs), walnut, and wheat germ oils (all high in omega-3 EFAs). And don't forget to *refrigerate!*

- The worst? Canola, corn, and soy oils (all genetically modified).

Healthy Fatty-Acid, Low-Glycemic Foods

- Dried beans, such as great northern, kidney, navy, and pinto are the healthiest low-glycemic food choices. A family that eats these beans regularly can meet all its EFA needs. Avoid corn and soy, however. Unless specifically labeled as organic and non-GMO, they are genetically modified and pumped full of viruses and antibiotics, as well as highly pesticide-laden foods.

- Coldwater fish, such as cod, haddock, halibut, herring, mackerel, salmon, or sea bass, are excellent.

FUNCTIONS AND SOURCES OF NUTRIENTS

Nutrient	Function	Sources
Proteins	Growth and maintenance	Goat milk, legumes, meat, poultry
Carbohydrates	Primary fuel source	Whole grains, fruits, vegetables
Fats and EFAs	Hormone production fuel source, cell membrane	Avocadoes, olives, raw nuts, seeds and their oils, and nut butters
Fiber	Digestive function, may prevent some diseases	Fruit, legumes, vegetables, whole grains
Cholesterol	Cell membranes, hormones, neurotransmitters	Eggs, meat, shellfish, healthy fats
Amino Acids	Protein synthesis, hormones, neural substances	Whey, eggs, coldwater fish, legumes, meat, poultry, whole grains
Vitamin A	Maintenance of bone and teeth, vision	Cheese, liver, milk (goat), vegetables
Vitamin B$_6$	Metabolism	Bananas, fish, legumes, nuts, poultry, whole grains
Vitamin D	Bone maintenance	BGH-free organic milk, fish-liver oil, sunshine
Vitamin C	Maintenance and repair of tissue and organs	Cabbage, cantaloupe, citrus, tomatoes
Folic Acid	Metabolism	Beans, dark-green leafy vegetables, liver, raw nuts
Niacin	Metabolism	Whole grains, lean meats, legumes
Pantothenic Acid	Metabolism	Widely distributed in foods
Riboflavin	Metabolism	Goat and sheep milks and cheeses, meats
Thiamin	Metabolism	Legumes, organ meats, whole grains
Calcium	Bone and teeth maintenance and growth	Broccoli, greens, sardines, almonds, goat's milk and cheese
Iron	Blood cell function	Dark-green leafy vegetables, eggs, legumes, meat, whole grains
Magnesium	Cell function	Bananas, beans, dark-green leafy vegetables, meat, nuts, poultry, whole grains
Phosphorus	Bone and teeth, kidney function, balance nerve and muscle function	Fruit, meat, asparagus, eggs, raw seeds and nuts, garlic
Zinc	Digestive enzymes, increases immunity	Beans, poultry, shellfish, whole grains, lamb, pecans, egg yolks

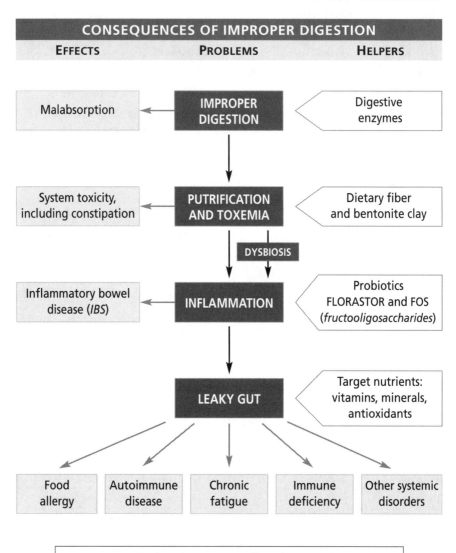

CONSEQUENCES OF IMPROPER DIGESTION

EFFECTS	PROBLEMS	HELPERS
Malabsorption	IMPROPER DIGESTION	Digestive enzymes
System toxicity, including constipation	PUTRIFICATION AND TOXEMIA	Dietary fiber and bentonite clay
	DYSBIOSIS	
Inflammatory bowel disease (IBS)	INFLAMMATION	Probiotics FLORASTOR and FOS (fructooligosaccharides)
	LEAKY GUT	Target nutrients: vitamins, minerals, antioxidants

Food allergy • Autoimmune disease • Chronic fatigue • Immune deficiency • Other systemic disorders

Animal or plant enzymes (fungal enzymes)
help with increased nutrient uptake as well as excretion of toxins.

THE TOP EIGHT FOOD ALLERGENS FOR MOST PEOPLE MOST OF THE TIME

DAIRY

• A high allergen, lactose gives milk its sweetness while casein is an exaggerated protein molecule that generally irritates and inflames the intestines.

WHEAT/GLUTEN

• Wheat is bleached with mercury-based solutions.
• Gluten is the sticky protein (makes up pudgy) found in most grains, such as pasta, the slurp of oatmeal when stirred, and the stickiness of white rice on your fingers when touched.

(*Try throwing a cooked noodle against a wall. It sticks. That's gluten.*)

SOY

• Generally high in genetically modified organisms (GMOs).
• High in viruses.

CORN

• Generally high in GMOs. Eat only organic, if possible.
• Abundantly sprayed with carcinogenic pesticides. Increases risk of breast cancer and diabetes.

SUGAR

• Suppresses immunity. Increases arterial and brain plaque and the risk of developing diabetes.

EGGS

• I really don't have the heart to condemn an egg. It is the "perfect" protein, but eat two to three time per week, not daily.

CITRUS

• Increases fermentation and mucus.

PEANUTS

• Very moldy—an increasingly common allergen. If you can't live without, consume no more than one to two times per month.

TOP TEN FOOD ADDITIVES TO AVOID

• **Aspartame.** This chemical sweetener has the longest list of complaints the Food and Drug Administration (FDA) has received. Aspartame also goes under such brand names as NutraSweet and Equal. Symptoms range from headaches, insomnia, mild depression, nausea, rashes, ringing ears, or vertigo to blurred vision, blindness, change of taste, loss of motor control, memory loss, slurred speech, suicidal depression, or seizures. Many doctors now warn pregnant women to avoid any products containing aspartame.

• **Brominated vegetable oil (BVO).** BVO is a potentially dangerous additive for some people. BVO is used as an emulsifier in foods and as a clouding agent in many popular soft drinks. Bromate, the main ingredient of BVO, is a poison—just one to four ounces of a 2-percent solution of BVO can severely poison a child.

- **Butylated hydroxyanisole (BHA), butylated hydroxytoluene (BHT), and tertiary butyhydroquinone (TBHQ).** All of these are chemicals used to prevent fats, oils, and container foods from becoming rancid. BHA or BHT are also often added to food-packaging materials. Researchers report that BHA in the diet of pregnant women results in brain enzyme changes in their offspring, including 50 percent decreased activity in brain choline, which is responsible for the transmission of nerve impulses. In animal studies, BHA and BHT also affect sleep, levels of depression, and weight. The authors of the research speculate that BHA and BHT can also affect the normal sequence of neurological development in young animals, too. Many consumers eat nearly 20 milligrams or more of BHA and BHT daily. Babies who are beginning to eat solid foods are estimated to ingest as much as 8 milligrams per day.

- TBHQ is often used along with BHA and BHT to spray the insides of cereal and cheese packages. Found mainly in candy bars, baking sprays, and fast foods, it is toxic at extremely low doses, and *has been implicated in childhood behavioral problems.*

- **Citrus red dye no. 2.** Used to color orange skins, citrus red dye no. 2 is a probable carcinogen and may cause chromosomal damage. Some experts contend that this compound does not migrate from the orange skin into the pulp, but the FDA has recommended a ban. Its continued use should be one more reason to seek out organically grown foods.

- **Monosodium glutamate (MSG).** MSG is a flavor enhancer widely used in Asia and often found in fast food, processed food, and packaged food. Symptoms of sensitivity include flushing of the skin, headaches, heart palpitations, nausea, and tightness of the chest.

- **Nitrates.** Used as preservatives in cured meats, such as bacon, ham, and smoked fish, to prevent spoilage. Nitrites and nitrates form cancer-causing compounds known as nitrosamines in the gastrointestinal tract. They have been associated with cancer and birth defects.

- **Pesticides.** Known to alter endocrine function. More than 1,400 pesticides are licensed for use on food crops, and every year greater than 2.5 billion pounds are dumped on croplands, forests, fields, and lawns. These, along with 260 million more pounds of chemicals discharged into surface waters (lakes and rivers), 2 billion pounds of air emissions, and several thousand food additives, are added to our foods and more inadvertently slip into our food supply during harvesting, processing, and packaging. The average American eats about 124 pounds of additives a year. Source: *2002 Advanced Nutrition Publications.*

- **Saccharin.** Still widely used as an artificial sweetener, this additive is a possible human carcinogen. Every packet of Sweet 'n Low has 40 milligrams of saccharin. It is also used as a sweetener in soft drinks. Causes liver cancer in test animals.

- **Sulfur dioxide, sodium bisulfite, and sulfites.** These are used to preserve foods, such as dried fruits, to prevent them from drying and stiffening, and are also used on shrimp and frozen potatoes. The FDA has received hundreds of letters reporting adverse reactions in asthma sufferers who have consumed foods with sulfiting agents. An increasing number of deaths caused by acute reactions to sulfites have been reported to the FDA.

- **Yellow dye no. 6.** Used in candy and carbonated beverages, yellow dye no. 6 increases the number of kidney and adrenal gland tumors in rats. It may also cause chromosomal damage, as well as allergic reactions. It has been banned in Norway and Sweden.

Appendix B

Information on Water

THE IMPORTANCE OF YOUR BODY'S WATER REQUIREMENTS

Your body relies on fluids for many functions in the body. For example, fluids act as a transport medium for nutrients to go from one part of the body to another. They also act as a lubricant in saliva and for joints.

Water plays an important part in maintaining body temperature. It helps excrete wastes in the body through the production of urine. Water is so important to your body's functions that it is directly absorbed in the stomach and reabsorbed in the large intestine. Water helps to flush the fat.

The chemical composition of water is H_2O. This means there are two hydrogen atoms for every oxygen atom contained in a molecule of water. The hydrogen is used in the body to help maintain the pH of the blood.

How Much Water Do You Need on a Daily Basis?

To calculate the amount of water you need every day multiply your weight by .075. This gives you the approximate number of 8-ounce cups needed by your body daily. Build up to drinking this amount gradually.

How Can You Get Water into Your Body?

- 3 cups of water can come from foods.
  - Whole grains contain 36 percent water.
  - Eggs contain 74 percent.

- Fruits and vegetables are great sources of water, as they contain 90 percent.
- Goat's milk contains 87 percent.
- Sheep and goat cheese contain 40 percent.
- $1\frac{1}{2}$ cups of water can come from the breakdown of food in your body.
- 8 cups of fluids, minimum, can come from pure water sources or herbal, nonsweetened teas.

To maintain the proper amount of water for all your body functions, you must have the same amount of water going in that goes out. Insufficient water results in cellular dehydration.

Under conditions of heavy athletic stress, a loss of 4–8 cups of water an hour is common. This is why it is so important for athletes in marathons or triathlons to consume fluids during competition.

What Type of Water is Best?

Pure water devoid of bacteria, chemicals, poisonous substances, and organic material is best. To date, I've found Fiji, Iceland, and Trinity to be the cleanest bottled waters. For tap water, the purification process of UV light and filtration, along with reverse osmosis, is most efficient in removing and reducing the widest range of contaminants. (*See* Preferred Bottled Water Suggestions in this appendix.)

CALCULATE YOUR BODY'S DAILY WATER REQUIREMENTS

Use this equation to calculate your daily requirements of water in cups:

Weight $\times$ .075 = The *minimum* number of cups of water per day

To convert the cups of water you require daily to ounces, use this equation:

Number of 8-ounce cups required $\times$ 8 ounces
= Total ounces of water required daily

Note: 16 cups = 128 ounces = 1 gallon, while 6 cups = 48 ounces = approximately 1 liter.

Some other important considerations about water include:

- For every glass of alcohol, coffee, soda, and the like that you consume, add an additional 8-ounce glass of water to your daily intake. These products are all diuretics and will increase dehydration.

- If you are currently drinking less than half your body's water requirements, you may want to increase your water consumption by one 8-ounce cup a week. While your body greatly needs this increase, it also needs time to adjust to the increase.

- Should you experience continued excessive urination, consider taking a multi-mineral (two, 3 times a day) after breakfast, lunch, and dinner. Good labels are Biotics, Douglas Labs, and Metagenics. For product information go to www.healingquestcenter.com.

Best Bottled Water Brands

1. Trinity   2. Fiji   3. Naya   4. Iceland

Remember: Glass bottles are always best! *Another mark of a better water is a low TDS count* (see the table below).

PREFERRED BOTTLED WATER SUGGESTIONS		
BRAND	SPRING LOCATION	TDS* (Below 500 is best)
Natural		
Chippewa Falls	Wisconsin	92
Arrowhead Spring	California	103
Naya	Canada	112
Mountain Valley	Arkansas	205
Hinckley Springs	Illinois	450
Perrier	France	505
Evian	France	562
Crystal Geyser	California	590
Pellegrino	Italy	1,180
Processed (locally filtered municipal source)		
Spring Valley		39
Hinckley Schmitt		60–70

*Total dissolved solvents, or heavy toxic metals

Note: For a referral to people who test water at no charge in your home, call the EPA Safe Drinking Water Hotline at 1-800-426-4791 or go to www.epa.gov/safewater.

Appendix C

Glycemic Index Information

GLYCEMIC INDEX BY FOOD CATEGORY			
FOOD CATEGORY	GLYCEMIC INDEX (%) 60% OR LESS IS BEST	FOOD CATEGORY	GLYCEMIC INDEX (%) 60% OR LESS IS BEST
Grain, Cereal Products		Cornflakes	80
Bread (white)	69	Muesli	66
Bread (whole meal)	72	Porridge oats	49
Buckwheat	51	Shredded Wheat	67
Millet	71	Weetabix	75
Pastry	59	**Biscuits**	
Rice (brown)	66	Digestive	59
Rice (white)	72	Oatmeal	54
Spaghetti (rice)	42	Rich tea	65
Spaghetti (wheat)	80	Ryvita	69
Sponge cake	46	Water	63
Sweet corn	82	**Sugars**	
Breakfast Cereals		Fructose	20
All-Bran	51	Glucose	100

Food Category	Glycemic Index (%) 60% or less is best	Food Category	Glycemic Index (%) 60% or less is best
Maltose	105	**Dried and Tinned Legumes**	
Sucrose	50	Beans (tinned, baked)	40
Miscellaneous		Beans (butter)	36
Fish fingers	38	Beans (haricot)	31
Honey	87	Beans (kidney)	29
Lucozade	95	Beans (soya)	15
Mars Bar	68	Beans (tinned soya)	14
Peanuts	13	Peas (blackeyed)	33
Potato crimps	51	Peas (chick)	36
Sausages	28	Peas (marrowfat)	47
Tomato soup	38	Lentils	29
Fresh Legumes		**Fruit**	
Broad beans	79	Apples (golden delicious)	39
Frozen peas	51	Bananas	82
Root Vegetables		Oranges	40
Beetroot	64	Raisins	64
Carrots	92	**Dairy Products***	
Parsnips	97	Ice cream	36
Potato (instant)	80	Milk (skimmed)	32
Potato (new)	70	Milk (whole)	34
Turnips	72	Yogurt	36
Yam	51		

Note: Only 25 gram carbohydrate portions given.

*Organic dairy is best as cow products contain lots of growth hormones that plump up body fat.

Source: Jenkins et al. *American Journal of Clinical Nutrition.* Vol 76, 1981.

To reduce the total glycemic index of a food, combine with a second food that is lower on the scale. Add the two values together then divide by 2 to obtain the Final Value. For example, raw almonds have a glycemic index of 0 and a banana has a glycemic index of 82. So the combined glycemic index of a snack of raw almonds and banana would look like this:

$$(0 + 82) \div 2 = 41 \text{ GI}$$

A snack of banana (82 GI) and raw nut butter (9 GI) would have the following glycemic index:

$$(82 + 9) \div 2 = 91 \div 2 = 45.5 \text{ GI}$$

While foods such as ice cream have a low glycemic index, it must be remembered that they also have a high saturated-fat content. Therefore, their total saturated-fat caloric value has to be considered, in addition to their possible long-term negative effect on insulin response.

GLYCEMIC INDEX OF CARBOHYDRATES					
LOW GLYCEMIC		MODERATE	HIGH		
Apples	Greens	Beets	Bagels	Breads:	Alcohol
Asparagus	Kiwi	Brown rice	Banana	whole wheat	Coffee
Broccoli	Peaches	Legumes	Carrots	white (Italian)	(regular
Cauliflower	Pears	Peas	Cereal	Desserts	& decaf)
Citrus	Peppers	Squash	Corn	Low-fat snacks	Soda
Grapes	Plums	Sweet potato	Melon	White potato	(regular
Green beans	Zucchini	Wild rice	Muffins	White rice	& decaf)
			Pasta	White sugar	
10–20%	20–30%	45–65%	80% – 90%		OFF THE CHART!
GOOD! ⟵			⟶ VERY HIGH		
Thigh Thinning, Insulin Regulating			Fat Storing, Thigh Plumpers		

Note: Healthy PUFA fatty acid foods are under 4%.

HEALTHY LOW-GLYCEMIC SHOPPING LIST

Protein Powders

❏ Pea, quinoa, rice, whey, vegetables

Fruits

❏ Apples (sour)
❏ Apricots (fresh)
❏ Blueberries
❏ Cherries
❏ Figs (fresh)
❏ Grapes
❏ Huckleberries
❏ Kiwis
❏ Kumquats
❏ Lemon juice
❏ Loganberries
❏ Mangos
❏ Mixed berries
❏ Mulberries
❏ Peaches
❏ Pears
❏ Prunes

Non-Wheat Carbohydrates

Seek low-gluten alternative breads, cereals, chips, crackers, and pastas

❏ Amaranth
❏ Brown rice
❏ Kamut
❏ Millet
❏ Quinoa
❏ Spelt
❏ Sprouted wheat
❏ Wild rice
❏ Legumes, squash, yams

Vegetables

❏ Artichokes
❏ Asparagus
❏ Bamboo shoots
❏ Okra
❏ Beans, green and yellow
❏ Beet tops
❏ Bok choy
❏ Broccoflower
❏ Broccoli
❏ Brussels sprouts
❏ Cauliflower
❏ Celery
❏ Chicory, red leaf
❏ Chives
❏ Collard greens
❏ Dandelion greens
❏ Endive
❏ Garlic
❏ Kale
❏ Kohlrabi
❏ Leeks
❏ Lettuce, Chinese
❏ Nappa cabbage
❏ Okra
❏ Onions
❏ Parsley
❏ Peppers, red, green, and yellow
❏ Sea vegetables (kelp, seaweed)
❏ Snow peas
❏ Spinach
❏ Squash
❏ Swiss chard
❏ Watercress
❏ Zucchini

EFAs—Healthy Oils and Foods

Do Not Heat:

❏ Essential Balance (my favorite!)
❏ Flaxseed oil, organic unrefined (kids only)
❏ Safflower oil
❏ Sunflower oil

Good for Cooking:

❏ Coconut oil
❏ Olive oil
❏ Ghee
❏ Sesame oil (organic, unrefined)

- ❏ Avocados and guacamole
- ❏ Hummus
- ❏ Olives
- ❏ Raw nut butters (almond, cashew, pumpkin)
- ❏ Rice/almond cheese
- ❏ Tapenades

Raw Nuts, Seeds, and Butters

- ❏ Almonds
- ❏ Cashews
- ❏ Filberts
- ❏ Macadamia
- ❏ Pecans
- ❏ Pistachios
- ❏ Pumpkin seeds
- ❏ Sesame seeds
- ❏ Sunflower seeds
- ❏ Walnuts

Coldwater Fish

No Tuna, Swordfish, Shark, or Warm Water Fish!

- ❏ Cod
- ❏ Haddock, wild
- ❏ Hake
- ❏ Halibut, wild
- ❏ Ocean char
- ❏ Sardines

- ❏ Salmon, wild
- ❏ Sea bass

Meats

- ❏ All free-range wild gamey meats
- ❏ Buffalo, duck, rabbit, pheasant, lamb
- ❏ Chicken or turkey sausage
- ❏ Free-range chicken (no antibiotics, hormones)
- ❏ Free-range turkey (no antibiotics, hormones)
- ❏ Lean beef (Roseland Farms, Faith in Place— my favorites*)

Natural Herbs and Spices

- ❏ Anise
- ❏ Basil
- ❏ Bay leaf
- ❏ Cardamom
- ❏ Cayenne (metabolism)
- ❏ Celery
- ❏ Cinnamon
- ❏ Cumin
- ❏ Dandelion
- ❏ Dill
- ❏ Fennel
- ❏ Garlic
- ❏ Ginger root
- ❏ Marjoram

- ❏ Mustard, dry
- ❏ Oregano
- ❏ Parsley
- ❏ Rosemary
- ❏ Saffron
- ❏ Savory
- ❏ Sea salt
- ❏ Tarragon
- ❏ Thyme
- ❏ Tumeric (good fat burner)

Preferred Beverages

No Distilled Water!

- ❏ Herbal teas
- ❏ Organic coffee (if you must)
- ❏ Ozonated spring water
- ❏ Reverse osmosis water

Kitchen Essentials

- ❏ Blender
- ❏ Broiler pan
- ❏ Coffee grinder (for nuts)
- ❏ Juicer (green juices best)
- ❏ Sauté pan (large)
- ❏ Sauté pan (medium)
- ❏ Sauté pan (small)
- ❏ Steamer
- ❏ Wok

*WEBSITES: *Roseland Farms: www.roselandfarms.com* • *Faith In Place: www.faithinplace.org*

INSULIN RESISTANCE AND LOW-CARBOHYDRATE DIETS

At first glance, insulin resistance (IR) seems a simple physiological imbalance. Insulin is simply unable to keep up with glucose, which is primarily derived from the breakdown of carbohydrates, causing elevated glucose to circulate in the blood, forcing more insulin to be released until the cells have been fed. While insulin helps feed the cells, it also signals the body to store excess carbohydrates in the form of adipose tissue (fat).

But IR is a more complex problem, creating multiple symptoms and concerns within the body. It is closely associated with Syndrome X or metabolic syndrome, conditions that can create abdominal obesity, blood fat disorders, or hypertension, and cause arterial plaque build-up. There may also be elevated C-reactive protein and homocysteine levels (which I recommend you test yearly through a blood workup), causing arterial inflammation and plaque build-up, early indicators for a heart attack.

High triglycerides, along with low HDL cholesterol, are prominent signs of Syndrome X. They are often overlooked or ignored until there is a major cardiac event. This cascade of symptoms can be traced back to elevated insulin.

The most common disorder associated with IR is a prediabetic condition. Because the signs and symptoms are ignored, IR can often develop into type 2 diabetes and brain disorders. Perhaps the most startling statistic comes from the American Diabetes Association, which has determined that more than 41 million Americans are in a prediabetic state of health.

The remedy for IR also appears simple—move to a low-glycemic/complex high-fiber carbohydrate, high PUFA (fatty-acid) diet. However, it is more complex than that. The presence of IR calls for a diet of complex high-fiber carbohydrates, certain proteins and fats, and the avoidance of other bad proteins, fats, and high-glycemic carbohydrates. Of course, it is critical to avoid sugars and simple carbohydrates, including pasta, white breads, white rice, and sugar. Complex carbohydrates, which are high in fiber, temper insulin rise and allow for longer periods of utilization of the carbohydrate energy while aiding digestion and scrubbing the liver. Most nonstarchy vegetables are acceptable for the diet, and these carbohydrates should account for 20 to 25 percent of the daily caloric intake.

Certain proteins should be avoided, including fast-food meats, high-fat red meats, and pork. The most ideal protein source to consider is mid-sized coldwater fish because it contains eicosapentaenoic acid (EPA), one of the most important fat sources to combat IR. This essential fatty acid improves insulin receptor-sites uptake at the same time it manufactures and repairs cell membranes, enabling the cells to obtain optimum nutrition and expel waste products. EPA also helps to decrease triglycerides, improve HDL levels, and provide anti-inflammatory action, which is important for anyone with metabolic syndrome.

Note: You must load up with omega-6 fatty acids (gamma linoleic acid [GLA]) for three to four weeks before adding EPA/DHA supplements to your regime. When supplementing with EFA fish oils, you should take a four-to-one ration of omega-6 (GLA) to omega-3 (fish oil).

Ideal choices of proteins to consume are bison, chicken (organic free range), loin of lamb, skinless duck, and turkey (also organic free range, if available). Try to sidestep highly saturated fat proteins. Foods high in healthy fats include avocados, hummus, olives, raw nuts, seeds, and oils from these foods. Many low-glycemic fruits, such as apples, berries, grapes, kiwis, peaches, pears, and plums, are acceptable.

An excellent food source to combat IR is the mistakenly maligned avocado. Avocados contain high-quality essential fats and proteins that are easily digested. Because of their low sugar content and absence of starch, avocados are excellent for people with diabetes or sugar-sensitive disorders, particularly at night as a bedtime snack. Interestingly, a good reason to consume avocados is their unique special sugar, known as mannoheptulose, which possesses the physiological ability to help the body control excess secretion of insulin.

You can also combat insulin resistance with daily exercise. While not technically an illness, IR is simply a serious sign of up-and-coming difficult and trying health issues.

FACTORS THAT HAVE BEEN OBSERVED TO AFFECT BLOOD GLUCOSE LEVELS

Substances and Other Factors	Increase	Decrease
Analgesic and Anti-Inflammatory		
Aspirin and salicylates/steroids	X	
Indomethacin	X	
Oxyphenbutazone		X
Phenylbutazone		X
Phenyramldol		X
Anti-Coagulants		
Bishydroxycoumarin		X
Antibiotics and Antibacterials		
Chloramphenicol		X
PAS and INH		X
Sulfonamides		X
Diuretics		
Thiazides	X	
Hormones		
ACTH	X	
Adrenal corticoids	X	
Androgen	X	
Growth hormone	X	
Epinephrine	X	
Estrogen	X	
Glucagon	X	
Oral contraceptives	X	
Thyroid	X	
Sedatives		
Barbiturates		X
Stimulants		
Caffeine	X	
Vasoactive Agents		
Epinephrine (Adrenalin)	X	
Propranolon HCL	X	

Substances and Other Factors	Increase	Decrease
Tranquilizers and Antidepressants		
Chlorpromazine	X	
MAO inhibitors		X
Miscellaneous		
Alcohol		X
Marijuana	X	
Nicotine	X	
Nicotinic acid (high dose)	X	
Probenecid		X
Pyribenzamine		X
Thiouracil (propylthiouracil)		X
Other Factors		
Antacidity	X	
Arthritis	X	
Coffee	X	
Gastrectomy	X	
Hypertension	X	
Jejunectomy	X	
Nephritis	X	
Obesity	X	
Prolonged inactivity	X	
Smoking	X	
Strenuous exercise		X
Stress		
Emotional	X	
Fever		X
Infection	X	
Physical injury		X
Pregnancy	X	
Surgery		X
Nutrition		
Fasting	X	
Overfeeding	X	
Starvation followed by refeeding	X	

Appendix D

All About Amino Acids

THE LIVER AND AMINO-ACID METABOLISM

Whether the source is protein, protein hydrolysates, di- and tripeptides, or singular amino acids, only singular amino acids enter the portal circulation. Portal circulation refers to the circulation of blood from the small intestine to the liver, via the portal vein.

Before entering the systemic circulation, which supplies nourishment to all of the tissue located throughout your body, with the exception of the heart and lungs because they have their own systems, amino acids must pass through the liver, the primary site of regulation for all the amino acids except the three branched-chain amino acids (BCAA: L-isoleucine, L-leucine, and L-valine). The primary site of BCAA metabolism is skeletal muscle.

The liver regulates the amount of essential amino acids entering the systemic circulation (other than BCAA) by increasing their breakdown only after the body's requirement for a particular amino acid is already achieved. Liver breakdown of nonessential amino acids increases progressively with rising intake.

Regulation by the liver, though, does not completely keep excess amino acids from entering the systemic circulation. The degree of regulation is also species dependent. The human liver, unlike that of animals, allows more of the dietary amino acids to enter the plasma. Consequently, in humans, plasma amino-acid levels correlate well with their dietary intake of proteins and/or amino acids. This correlation allows for greater manipulation of plasma amino-acid levels, which can potentially provide therapeutic effects.

What does all this mean? You must eat a wide variety of protein/amino acid-bearing foods. It is not healthy to consume *just chicken* every day. If you do, you will not derive all the essential amino acids necessary to support brain, muscle, nerves, and metabolism.

THE BRAIN AND AMINO-ACID METABOLISM

The brain requires a constant environment in order to function properly. This environment is maintained by the blood-brain barrier (BBB). Covering 99.5 percent of the capillary surface of the brain, this anatomical barrier regulates the flow of nutrients between the brain and systemic circulation.

The BBB performs its regulatory function through various transport systems that determine what goes in and out of the brain. Among the many substances regulated are amino acids. Different types of amino acids have different transport systems, but the most important is the one that transports the large neutral amino acids (LNAA), such as isoleucine, leucine, phenylalanine, tryptophan, tyrosine, and valine. Since all of these amino acids utilize the same transport system, they are all competing for entry into the brain (hence a happy brain).

Increasing the ratio of one of the LNAA amino acids relative to the others increases the entry of that particular amino acid into the brain. Measuring a person's LNAA ratio can, therefore, help predict therapeutic response.

Amino Acid Therapy

The effectiveness of amino acid therapy can be greatly influenced by when and how amino acids are administered. This simple variable is one explanation for the discrepancies in the results of various studies. This is why measuring plasma urine amino-acid levels provides helpful information in determining and justifying treatment in various neurochemical disorders, such as depression, ALS (amyotrophic lateral sclerosis), and Parkinson's disease to name a few. Each grouping may suggest deficiencies of one or a number of amino acids in certain disease conditions. So it's extremely important that you rotate your proteins on a daily basis. To recap, high quality amino-acid based proteins such as whey, eggs, coldwater fish, legumes, meat, poultry, and organic whole grains are all high in amino acids. Always consider attaining the full spectrum of nine essential amino acids and supplement daily if you are vegetarian or your protein choices are repetitive.

AMINO ACID GROUP	MAJOR AREA OF NEED
Neurotransmitter Amino Acids	
Asparagine	
Aspartic acid	Anxiety/stress
G-aminobutyric acid (GABA)	Brain
Glutamic acid	Depression
Glutamine	Drug dependency
Phenylalanine*	Heart
Taurine	Insomnia
Tryptophan*	
Tyrosine	
Branched-Chain Amino Acids	
Arginine	Bone health
Isoleucine*	Exercise
Leucine*	Injury
Valine*	Muscle wasting
	Surgery
Sulfur-Containing Amino Acids	
Cysteine	Allergies
Homocysteine	Chemo/radiation
Methionine*	Skin health
Taurine	
Aspartic acid	Chronic fatigue
	Stamina
Lysine*	
Histidine*	
Threonine*	

Indicates the nine essential amino acids. They must be obtained from a variety of different protein sources, preferably organic, non-GMO, and hormone-free.

Appendix E

The Gift of the Glandulars

THE THYROID

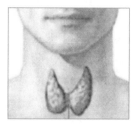

The thyroid gland is a soft, small, bow-shaped gland. It comprises a right and left lobe bridged with tissue called the isthmus, which joins the two lobes. The thyroid is located in the neck below the voice box (larynx) and is situated on either side of the windpipe (trachea).

HOW DOES YOUR THYROID WORK?

Most thyroid tissue consists of follicular cells that secrete iodine-containing hormones called thyroxine (T4) and tri-iodothyronine (T3). The parafollicular cells secrete the hormone calcitonin. The thyroid needs iodine to produce the hormones.

The thyroid gland is controlled by TSH (thyroid stimulating hormone), which is secreted by the pituitary gland at the base of the brain. TSH travels through the blood to stimulate the production of thyroxine (T4 hormone from your thyroid gland). T4 controls your metabolism. If there is not enough T4, your body will slow down and you become hypothyroid. If you have too much T4, your body will speed up and you will become hyperthyroid.

- According to the Thyroid Gland entry of the *Endocrinology Health Guide* at www.umm.edu regarding the functions of the thyroid gland: "The thyroid plays an important role in regulating the body's metabolism and calcium balance. The T4 and T3 hormones stimulate every tissue in the body to produce proteins and increase the amount of oxygen used by cells. The harder the cells work, the harder the organs work. The calcitonin hormone works together with the parathyroid hormone to regulate calcium levels in the body."

- Levels of hormones secreted by the thyroid are controlled by the pituitary gland's thyroid-stimulating hormone, which in turn is controlled by the hypothalamus. I refer to the pituitary and hypothalamus as the happy, depression, and anxiety centers of the brain.

- Predisposition to low thyroid or thyroid disease can occur with the following conditions:

  - autoimmune problem—you can develop Hashimoto's thyroiditis or Graves' disease (saliva adrenal testing recommended)
  - iodine deficiency
  - long-term fatty-acid deficiency
  - multi-mineral, B and C vitamin deficiencies
  - potassium-iodide deficiency—lump(s) can form in or on the gland
  - years of insult due to high levels of non-stop stress
  - years of going to sleep long past 10 P.M.
  - Years of sub-optimal calorie intake

  (Adapted from an article by the Australian Thyroid Foundation, Ltd.)

THYROIDITIS

Thyroiditis is a common condition that can enlarge and inflame the thyroid gland. There are a number of forms of thyroiditis, but the most common type is Hashimoto's thyroiditis, or hyperthyroidism.

HYPERTHYROIDISM

Hyperthyroidism is a result of your thyroid speeding up. This may occur over a period of time. Generally, after years of low thyroid function, or hypothyroidism, your thyroid leaps into hyperthyroidism in an attempt to jumpstart your system. Hyperthyroidism is considered the last phase of destruction before the thyroid gives up and stops producing hormones. I recommend pure fish-oil sources, such as cod liver oil on an empty stomach, to halt the progression. Amounts will vary depending on blood values and weight. **Note:** Excessive long-term intake of cod liver oil can lower thyroid function too much.

Hyperthyroidism changes may be subtle or marked, depending on what stage the disease has developed in the body. The most common form of hyperthyroidism is Graves' disease, which is generally reversible.

The Most Common Symptoms of Hyperthyroidism

- anxiety
- diarrhea or frequent bowel movements
- eye problems
- heat intolerance
- heart disease
- hyperactivity
- muscle weakness
- palpitations/racing heart
- sex hormone imbalances
- weight loss

HYPOTHYROIDISM

Hypothyroidism is a result of your system slowing down. This may occur over a period of time. In hypothyroidism, changes are subtle and sometimes difficult to diagnose accurately.

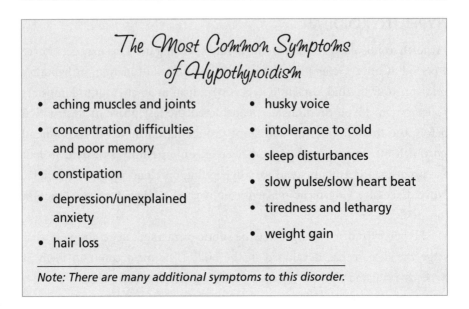

The Most Common Symptoms of Hypothyroidism

- aching muscles and joints
- concentration difficulties and poor memory
- constipation
- depression/unexplained anxiety
- hair loss

- husky voice
- intolerance to cold
- sleep disturbances
- slow pulse/slow heart beat
- tiredness and lethargy
- weight gain

Note: There are many additional symptoms to this disorder.

Test for Hypothyroidism: Armpit Temperature Log

There is considerable evidence that the current tests for the diagnosis of hypothyroidism (low thyroid function) are insensitive and somewhat lacking in accuracy.

In his book, *Hypothyroidism: The Unsuspected Illness*, endocrinologist and thyroid specialist Broda Barnes, M.D., explains his feelings and theories about this matter. He proposes that the most sensitive and accurate test for picking up the highest percentage of people with low thyroid function is simply to check the most basic function of the thyroid—it's ability to regulate the metabolic furnace of the body, that is, to create heat or control temperature. Dr. Barnes feels that recording basal body temperature daily for ten days is the simplest and best means of doing this. For accuracy, he insists that the person be absolutely relaxed.

Instructions for Recording Basal Body Temperature

1. Use a basal or oral thermometer that has been shaken down the night before and put on your bedside stand.

2. Put the thermometer under your armpit (ten minutes for a mercury thermometer, ten to thirty seconds for a digital thermometer). Record your armpit temperature each morning for ten days (use the table provided on page 132). Do this before you've gotten out of bed, urinated, had coffee, or had any activity, mental or physical. Dr. Barnes suggests using the auxiliary (armpit) temperature rather than the mouth, as a large number of people have low-grade unsuspected sinus infections, which can generate heat in the mouth, thereby falsely raising the oral temperature.

3. For women, additional considerations are needed. During ovulation, your temperature is generally somewhat elevated, so women who menstruate should start recording on the second or third day of their cycle. (For menopausal or post-menopausal women, it makes no difference which day of the month is tested.) Normal armpit temperature is 97.6 degrees Fahrenheit. One degree below this value indicates a 13-percent decrease in basal metabolic rate (BMR), indicating lowered thyroid and adrenal function.

This temperature-recording data generally correlates with your blood thyroid hormone levels (when evaluated), a thermogram (where available), and your thyroid history questionnaire sheet. Hypothyroidism is a common and easily treatable ailment. Barnes estimates that approximately 40 percent of the adult population has this problem and says that it can be associated with acne, allergies, depression, hypertension, hypoglycemia, obesity, psoriasis, and undiagnosed skin problems, plus a host of other ailments. If you have any of these unusual reactions, please indicate them on the recording sheet.

Begin by consuming enough calories daily, increase your percentage of EFAs to 50 percent of your total daily calorie requirement, and—*lights out by 10 P.M.; stop all monkey business and go to sleep!* You should begin to see small incremental increases in your armpit temperature within the next one to three months.

Copy and use the Armpit Temperature Chart below. It's an important tool in your quest for healthy living and burning fat.

ARMPIT TEMPERATURE LOG

Name_____ Date _____

RECORD DATE	# HOURS OF SLEEP	TIME YOU GO TO SLEEP	TIME YOU WAKE UP	MORNING TEMPERATURE
1				
2				
3				
4				
5				
6				
7				
8				
9				
10				
11				
12				
13				
14				

ADRENAL GLANDS AND YOUR CORTISOL CLOCK

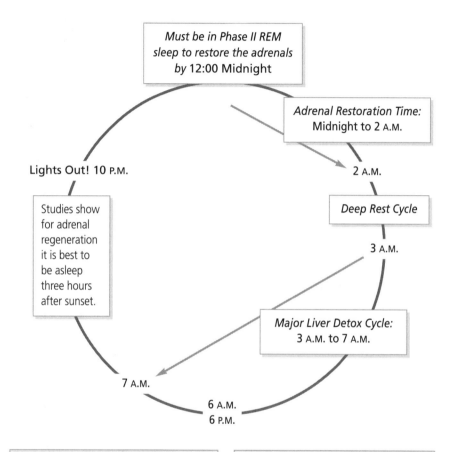

Must be in Phase II REM sleep to restore the adrenals by 12:00 Midnight

Adrenal Restoration Time: Midnight to 2 A.M.

Lights Out! 10 P.M.

2 A.M.

Studies show for adrenal regeneration it is best to be asleep three hours after sunset.

Deep Rest Cycle

3 A.M.

Major Liver Detox Cycle: 3 A.M. to 7 A.M.

7 A.M.

6 A.M.
6 P.M.

1. If you are not sleeping by 10 P.M., in Phase II REM sleep by midnight, your adrenals cannot be *fixed* for you to get up for the great fight of life the following day.

2. If you do not honor your adrenal restoration cycle, your body cannot adequately detox from 3 to 7 A.M. Hence, you keep stacking your toxins day after day, month after month, year after year. This is termed your **Total Toxic Load** or **Body Burden**.

Tampers with Adrenal Function
- Not going to bed early enough
- Not sleeping 8.5 hours
- Disturbed sleep
- Not enough calories daily
- High dead-food dietary choices
- Over-consumption of:
  - Coffee/soda   ∘ Sugar
  - Alcohol   ∘ Medications
- Low PUFA fat, multi-minerals vitamin C and B-complex intake

Creating Clarity About Colonics

A colon irrigation, preferably using the nonpressurized gravitational method (which is gentle and ideal), is an internal bath that helps cleanse the colon of poisons, gas, and years of accumulated fecal matter. Unlike an enema, it does not involve the retention of water. There is little to no discomfort or internal pressure, just a steady gentle flow of water in and out of the colon.

When a person receives a colonic, he/she lies on a warmed table. A sterilized speculum is gently inserted into the rectum. Water flow is always under direct control of the practitioner. It flows into the colon via a small water tube and out through the evacuation tube, carrying with it impacted feces, mucous, and toxins.

As the water flows out of the colon, the practitioner gently massages the abdomen and specific meridians to help the colon release its contents. It is possible to see this expelled waste matter when it passes through a special viewing window in the evacuation tank. Each client is well covered and modesty is given top priority during the procedure. This closed colonic method takes only thirty to forty minutes.

The number of treatments will always vary with the individual, given the condition of her/his health. Often, the waste is so hard and firmly lodged in the colon that it may take a series of colonics to sufficiently soften and loosen this accumulated fecal material. Some people may not have desired results for the first few treatments, which is why a series of treatments is often necessary and advisable. Colonic irrigation is most effective when employed in combination with ample water intake, exercise, and a high-fiber diet consisting of nonmucous-producing foods. Fresh fruits, vegetables, and certain herbs and oils are suggested to help loosen and dissolve accumulated fecal matter.

The suggested series for a detoxification is two colonics a week for eight weeks. Once the colon is clean, it is advisable to have a colonic every one to two months to maintain an optimal internal environment. Detoxification utilizing colonics is recommended at the change of seasons when diet and exercise patterns often change. Always consider a colonic before, during, and after a fast to hasten the removal of toxic debris. Colonics are also very beneficial during the cold and flu season.

Colonics offer relief from a variety of disturbances by cleansing the colon of impacted and putrefactive fecal matter. People have found relief through the use of colon cleansing for many conditions, including cold hands and feet, fatigue, gas, headaches, irritability, lethargy, and skin problems. Constipation and chronic diarrhea can also be alleviated. Your sense of well-being is often dramatically improved with colon irrigation. Typically, you feel lighter and more energetic. The body can once again assimilate food in the colon and better defend itself against disease. Natural peristalsis, muscle tone, and regularity are eventually restored, and many serious diseases may be averted through this gentle, sterile, scientific technique. Colonics are a key factor in the restoration of the body's natural balance, or what is termed good health.

There are virtually no side effects. People who are extremely toxic, however, may start to feel as though they have a cold or headache after a colonic. This is mainly because toxins that have been lying dormant in the colon are now being flushed out and a small amount of them may be reabsorbed into the system. This healing crisis passes quickly and is replaced by a feeling of well-being with further treatments.

Colonics will not damage normal intestinal flora. One function of the first half of the colon is to create intestinal flora needed for the colon. When the accumulation of feces in the bowel leads to fecal encrustation, it is difficult for the colon to function normally, and the villi in this lining cannot

Appendix G

Daily Food Logs

HOW TO USE THE DAILY FOOD LOGS

1. Each food log is a record of your entire daily food intake. Refer to the Explanatory Daily Food Log on pages 144–145 for a layout and key.

2. Logs should be read across, left to right, for components of each meal (Breakfast, Snack, Lunch, Dinner, etc.).

3. The 1200, 1700, and 2500 Calorie Food Logs on pages 146–151 are examples of how to achieve a thigh-thinning regimen on a daily basis. You should *not* begin any such program without medical or nutritional counseling.

4. The Blank Food Log provided on pages 152–153 will help you keep track of the amounts, percentages, and grams, plus the types of food you *actually* eat on a daily basis.

5. You may photocopy the Blank Food Log for re-use.

6. Food Logs for your particular *recommended* Daily Caloric Intake can be downloaded from the PRODUCTS page on our website at: www.Healing QuestCenter.com for 99 cents each through our PayPal link.

7. Practice! Practice! Practice!

EXPLANATORY DAILY FOOD LOG

NAME:

A →	PROTEIN		FAT	STARCHY CARBS*
U = unit	1 unit = 55 calories/7grams		1 unit = 22 calories/2.5 grams	1 unit = 40 calories/9 grams
Food Portion Examples **B**	1oz lean protein 2 egg whites / 1 whole egg 1.5 oz fish 1oz almond cheese 2 oz low-fat cottage cheese		3 olives / $^1/_3$ tsp olive oil 2 slices avocado OR $^1/_4$ cup guacamole 3 almonds / 1 tsp raw nuts $^1/_2$ tsp Essential Balance** oil OR organic sesame oil $^1/_2$ tsp raw nut butter	$^1/_2$ medium potato (sweet/yam) $^1/_2$ cup legumes $^1/_5$ cup brown rice $^1/_2$ slice non-wheat bread $^1/_2$ cup beets or peas or carrots
BREAKFAST	2U	← **C** →	8U	
Time:				
Snack			4U	
Time:				
LUNCH	2.5U		4U	1U
Time:				
Snack			4U	
Time:				
DINNER	2U		4U	1U
Time:				
Snack			3U	
Time:				
Units Goal	6.5U		27U	
% Calories Goal	30%		50%	
Calories Total	360		600	
Grams Total	46		68	
			Cooked oils do not count	Non-wheat is best

G — Units Goal / % Calories Goal
H — Calories Total / Grams Total

KEY

A The food groups included in each meal or snack (protein, fat, and starchy, veggie, and fruit carbohydrates).

B 1 single unit (U) portion or the value in grams or calories and examples; units vary by daily calorie intake allotted.

C The number of units (U) allotted under the food group listed.

D List any reactions noted when consuming certain foods.

E Record daily:
— number cups of water consumed
— armpit temperature taken before rising each morning
— total hours slept
— daily energy rating (10 is high)
— inches of BMs (should be 24" daily)

DATE:

VEGGIE CARBS*	FRUIT CARBS*	List Symptoms
1 unit = 25 calories/9 grams	1 unit = 30 calories/9 grams	*Avoid all dairy, corn, wheat, soy, citrus, caffeine, and refined sugar for first six weeks.*
2 cups raw veggies 2 cups crisp veggies 1 cup cooked, limp veggies 4 cups spinach/lettuce 12 oz fresh juice $^1/_2$ medium apple $^1/_2$ cup berries	1 cup strawberries 1 small kiwi or plum $^1/_2$ cup bottled juice	
	1U	
	1U	**D**
1U		
1U		
F		**E**
6–7U		Water (cups) _____
20%		Temperature (A.M.) _____
240		Sleep (hours) _____
63		Energy (1–10) _____
		BMs (inches) _____

F Combined totals of Starchy, Veggie, and Fruit carbs.

G Total *recommended* units & calories/grams allotted for each category daily; units vary by daily calorie intake allotted.

H Total calories/grams *actually* consumed daily; Calorie Total per group = Unit Goal achieved x 55 calories; Grams total per group = Unit Goal achieved x 7.

— 1 U of protein would be equal to 1oz lean protein or 2 oz low fat cottage cheese.

— If you consume 2 U's of protein you double the single portion size listed.

1200 CALORIE DAILY FOOD LOG

NAME:

	PROTEIN		**FAT**		**STARCHY CARBS***	
U = unit	1 unit = 55 calories/7 grams		1 unit = 22 calories/2.5 grams		1 unit = 40 calories/9 grams	
Food Portion Examples	1oz lean protein 2 egg whites / 1 whole egg 1.5 oz fish 1oz almond cheese 2 oz low-fat cottage cheese		3 olives / $^1/_3$ tsp olive oil 2 slices avocado OR $\quad ^1/_4$ cup guacamole 3 almonds / 1 tsp raw nuts $^1/_2$ tsp Essential Balance** oil $\quad$ OR organic sesame oil $^1/_2$ tsp raw nut butter		$^1/_2$ medium potato (sweet/yam) $^1/_2$ cup legumes $^1/_5$ cup brown rice $^1/_2$ slice non-wheat bread $^1/_2$ cup beets or peas or carrots	
BREAKFAST	**2U**		**8U**			
Time:	2 scoops protein powder $\quad$ = 14 grams protein - - - - - - - - - - - - - - - - OR 4 egg whites OR 2 oz chicken sausages		2 tsp EB oil + 2 tsp $\quad$ coconut oil - - - - - - - - - - - - - - - With 2 small avocados		In blender, mix all oils $\quad$ and vitamins with fiber $\quad$ and water - - - - - - - - - - - - - - - With $^1/_2$ slice toast	
Snack			**4U**			
Time:			2 tsp raw nut butter OR $\quad$ 12 large olives - - - - - - - - - - - - - - - OR $^1/_2$ small container $\quad$ hummus		- - - - - - - - - - - - - - - With 5 rice snap crackers	
LUNCH	**2.5U**		**4U**		**1U**	
Time:	2.5 oz animal protein OR 4 oz coldwater fish		2 tsp Essential Balance oil		$^1/_2$ cup corn or brown rice OR $^1/_2$ cup peas, carrots OR $^1/_2$ slice non-wheat bread	
Snack			**4U**			
Time:			4 tsp raw nuts OR 4 oz goat cheese			
DINNER	**2U**		**4U**		**1U**	
Time:	2 oz animal protein OR 3 oz coldwater fish		2 tsp Essential Balance oil		$^1/_2$ medium sweet potato OR $^1/_2$ cup legumes OR brown rice	
Snack			**3U**			
Time:			1 small avocado OR 9 large olives			
Units Goal	6.5U		27U			
% Calories Goal	30%		50%			
Calories Total	360		600			
Grams Total	46		68			
			Cooked oils do not count		Non-wheat is best	

Remarks: *Calorie total will vary based on type of carbohydrate consumed

DATE:			
VEGGIE CARBS*		**FRUIT CARBS***	**List Symptoms**
1 unit = 25 calories/9 grams		1 unit = 30 calories/9 grams	*Avoid all dairy, corn, wheat, soy, citrus, caffeine, and refined sugar for first six weeks.*
2 cups raw veggies 2 cups crisp veggies 1 cup cooked, limp veggies 4 cups spinach/lettuce 12 oz fresh juice $1/_2$ medium apple $1/_2$ cup berries		1 cup strawberries 1 small kiwi or plum $1/_2$ cup bottled juice	
		1U	
			With $1/_2$ cup frozen mixed organic berries OR $1/_3$ frozen banana
		1U	
			With small apple or pear OR 9 grapes, etc.
1U			
	2 cups lightly steamed veggies (Weeks 1 & 2 NO RAW for now)		
1U			
	2 cups steamed veggies OR 4 cups salad		
6–7U			Water (cups) _____
20%			Temperature (A.M.) _____
240			Sleep (hours) _____
63			Energy (1–10) _____
			BMs (inches) _____

**Essential Balance oil contains a balanced ratio of omega-3 and omega-6.*

1700 CALORIE DAILY FOOD LOG

NAME:

	PROTEIN		FAT	STARCHY CARBS*
U = unit	1 unit = 55 calories/7grams		1 unit = 22 calories/2.5 grams	1 unit = 40 calories/9 grams
Food Portion Examples	1oz lean protein 2 egg whites / 1 whole egg 1.5 oz fish 1oz almond cheese 2 oz low-fat cottage cheese		3 olives / $^1/_3$ tsp olive oil 2 slices avocado OR $^1/_4$ cup guacamole 3 almonds / 1 tsp raw nuts $^1/_2$ tsp Essential Balance** oil OR organic sesame oil $^1/_2$ tsp raw nut butter	$^1/_2$ medium potato (sweet/yam) $^1/_2$ cup legumes $^1/_5$ cup brown rice $^1/_2$ slice non-wheat bread $^1/_2$ cup beets or peas or carrots
BREAKFAST	2U		12U	
Time:	2 scoops protein powder = 14 grams protein OR - - - - - - - - - - - - - - - - - - 4 egg whites		1 Tbl Essential Balance oil + 1 Tbl coconut oil - - - - - - - - - - - - - - - - - - With 2 medium avocados	In blender, mix all oils and vitamins with fiber and water - - - - - - - - - - - - - - - - - - With $^1/_2$ slice toast
Snack			4U	
Time:			2 tsp raw nut butter OR - - - - - - - - - - - - - - - - - - 4 tsp raw nuts	
LUNCH	4U		6U	2U
Time:	4 oz animal protein OR 6 oz coldwater fish		1 Tbls Essential Balance oil OR 2 tsp. olive oil	1 slice non-wheat bread OR 1 cup beets, peas, carrots
Snack			6U	1U
Time:			1 small container hummus OR 18 large olives	6 organic corn chips OR 5 rice crackers
DINNER	3U		6U	2U
Time:	3 oz animal protein OR 4.5 oz coldwater fish		1 Tbls Essential Balance oil OR 2 tsp olive oil	1 medium sweet potato OR $^1/_2$ cup beans or brown rice, or corn
Snack			4U	
Time:			1 medium avocado	
Units Goal	9U		39U	
% Calories Goal	30%		50%	
Calories Total	510		850	
Grams Total	65		97	
			Cooked oils do not count	Non-wheat is best

*Remarks: *Calorie total will vary based on type of carbohydrate consumed*

DATE:			
VEGGIE CARBS*		**FRUIT CARBS***	**List Symptoms**
1 unit = 25 calories/9 grams		1 unit = 30 calories/9 grams	*Avoid all dairy, corn, wheat, soy, citrus, caffeine, and refined sugar for first six weeks.*
2 cups raw veggies 2 cups crisp veggies 1 cup cooked, limp veggies 4 cups spinach/lettuce 12 oz fresh juice $\frac{1}{2}$ medium apple $\frac{1}{2}$ cup berries		1 cup strawberries 1 small kiwi or plum $\frac{1}{2}$ cup bottled juice	
		1U	
		With $\frac{1}{2}$ cup frozen organic berries OR a small apple or pear -	
		1U	
		A small apple or pear - With 1 Tbls raisins	
1U			
	2 cups well- steamed veggies (Weeks 1 & 2 NO RAW for now)		
1U			
	2 cups well-steamed veggies		
10U			Water (cups) _____
20%			Temperature (A.M.) _____
340			Sleep (hours) _____
90			Energy (1–10) _____
			BMs (inches) _____

**Essential Balance oil contains a balanced ratio of omega-3 and omega-6.

2500 CALORIE DAILY FOOD LOG

NAME:

	PROTEIN		FAT	STARCHY CARBS*	
U = unit	1 unit = 55 calories/7grams		1 unit = 22 calories/2.5 grams	1 unit = 40 calories/9 grams	
Food Portion Examples	1oz lean protein 2 egg whites / 1 whole egg 1.5 oz fish 1oz almond cheese 2 oz low-fat cottage cheese		3 olives / $1/_3$ tsp olive oil 2 slices avocado OR $1/_4$ cup guacamole 3 almonds / 1 tsp raw nuts $1/_2$ tsp Essential Balance** oil OR organic sesame oil $1/_2$ tsp raw nut butter	$1/_2$ medium potato (sweet/yam) $1/_2$ cup legumes $1/_5$ cup brown rice $1/_2$ slice non-wheat bread $1/_2$ cup beets or peas or carrots	
BREAKFAST	**4U**		**12U**		
Time:		4 scoops protein powder = 21–28 grams protein OR - - - - - - - - - - - - - - - - - - 8 egg whites	1Tbls Essential Balance oil + 1Tbls coconut oil - - - - - - - - - - - - - - - - - - With 2 large avocados	In blender, mix all oils & vitamins with water - - - - - - - - - - - - - - - - - - With 1 slice toast	
Snack			**8U**		
Time:			4 tsp raw nut butter OR 6 tsp raw nuts		
LUNCH	**4U**		**12U**	**2U**	
Time:		5 oz animal protein OR 7.5 oz coldwater fish	2 Tbls Essential Balance oil OR 2 tsp. olive oil or coconut oil	1 slice non-wheat bread OR $1/_2$ cup brown rice OR $1/_2$ cup organic corn chips	
Snack			**8U**	**1U**	
Time:			$1^1/_3$ small container hummus OR 18 large olives	1 cup veggie sticks OR 5 rice crackers	
DINNER	**4U**		**8U**	**2U**	
Time:		4 oz animal protein OR 6 oz coldwater fish	1 Tbls Essential Balance oil OR 2 tsp olive oil	1 medium sweet potato OR $1/_2$ cup organic peas OR $1/_2$ cup legumes	
Snack			**8U**		
Time:			1 large avocado OR 24 large olives		
Units Goal	**13–14U**		**57U**		
% Calories Goal	**30%**		**50%**		
Calories Total	750		1,250		
Grams Total	98		142		
			Cooked oils do not count	**Non-wheat is best**	

Remarks: *Calorie total will vary based on type of carbohydrate consumed

DATE:			
VEGGIE CARBS*		**FRUIT CARBS***	**List Symptoms**
1 unit = 25 calories/9 grams		1 unit = 30 calories/9 grams	*Avoid all dairy, corn, wheat, soy, citrus, caffeine, and refined sugar for first six weeks.*
2 cups raw veggies 2 cups crisp veggies 1 cup cooked, limp veggies 4 cups spinach/lettuce 12 oz fresh juice $^1/_2$ medium apple $^1/_2$ cup berries		1 cup strawberries 1 small kiwi or plum $^1/_2$ cup bottled juice	
		2U	
			1 cup frozen organic berries OR small apple or pear
		2U	
			1 medium apple or pear
1U			
	2 cups well- steamed veggies (Weeks 1 & 2 NO RAW for now)		
		2U	
			1 medium fruit
1U			
	2 cups well-steamed veggies		
13–14U			Water (cups) _____
20%			Temperature (A.M.) _____
500			Sleep (hours) _____
128			Energy (1–10) _____
			BMs (inches) _____

**Essential Balance oil contains a balanced ratio of omega-3 and omega-6.

BLANK DAILY FOOD LOG

NAME:

	PROTEIN	FAT	STARCHY CARBS*
U = unit	1 unit = 55 calories/7grams	1 unit = 22 calories/2.5 grams	1 unit = 40 calories/9 grams
Food Portion Examples	1 oz lean protein 2 egg whites / 1 whole egg 1.5 oz fish 1 oz almond cheese 2 oz low-fat cottage cheese	3 olives / $\frac{1}{3}$ tsp olive oil 2 slices avocado or $\frac{1}{4}$ cup guacamole 3 almonds/1 tsp raw nuts $\frac{1}{2}$ tsp Essential Balance** oil / organic sesame oil $\frac{1}{2}$ tsp raw nut butter	$\frac{1}{2}$ medium potato (sweet / yam) $\frac{1}{4}$ cup legumes $\frac{1}{5}$ cup brown rice $\frac{1}{2}$ slice non-wheat bread $\frac{1}{2}$ cup beets or peas or carrots
BREAKFAST						
Time:						
Snack						
Time:						
LUNCH						
Time:						
Snack						
Time:						
DINNER						
Time:						
Snack						
Time:						
Units Goal						
% Calories Goal						
Calories Total						
Grams Total						
		Cooked oils do not count	Non-wheat is best	

Remarks: *Calorie total will vary based on type of carbohydrate consumed

References and Recommended Reading

Australian Thyroid Foundation, Ltd. Westmead NSW Australia. www.thyroid-foundation.com.au.

Barnes, Broda, M.D., and Galton, Lawrence. *Hypothyroidism: The Unsuspected Illness.* Toronto, CANADA: HarperCollins, Fitzhenry and Whiteside, Ltd., 1976.

Brand-Miller, J. "Revised International Table of Glycemic Index and Glycemic Load Values." *American Journal of Clinical Nutrition* (July 2002).

Dagenais, GR, Yi, Q, Mann, JFE, et al. "Prognostic impact of body weight and abdominal obesity in women and men with cardiovascular disease." *American Heart Journal* (January 2005): 54–60.

Ferrier, H, Nieuwenhuijsen, M, Boobis, A, et al. "Current knowledge and recent developments in consumer exposure assessment of pesticides: A UK perspective." *2002 Advanced Nutrition Publications* (September 2002):19.

Willett, Walter, Skerrett, PJ. *Eat, Drink, and Be Healthy: The Harvard Medical School Guide to Healthy Eating.* Cambridge, MA: The Free Press, 2005.

Wolever, TMS, Taylor, RH , et al. "Glycemic index of foods: a physiological basis." *American Journal of Clinical Nutrition* (July 2002): 286–289.

Young, LR. *The Portion Teller: Smartsize Your Way to Permanent Weight Loss.* New York, NY: Morgan Road Books, 2005.

RECOMMENDED READING

The following selection of articles, books, and websites have helped create the wealth of knowledge imparted in this book.

American Journal of Clinical Nutrition 2002 Glycemic Index at www.ajcn.org/cgi/content/full/76/1/5/T1.

Anderson, JW, Konz, EC, Jenkins, DJ. "Health Advantages and Disadvantages of Weight-Reducing Diets: A Computer Analysis and Critical Review." *Journal of the American College of Nutrition* 19(5). (2000).

Bland, J. (ed.). *Yearbook of Nutritional Medicine.* New Canaan, CT: Keats Publishing, Inc., 1985.

Daly, A, Delahanty, L, Wylie-Rosett, J. "101 weight loss tips for preventing and controlling diabetes." American Diabetes Association, 2003.

Davies, S, Stewart, A. *Nutritional Medicine.* London: Dan Books, 1987.

Drenowski, A, Kurth, C, Holden-Wiltse, J, et al. "Food preferences in human obesity: Carbohydrates versus fats." *Appetite* (1992): 18.

Erasmus, Udo. *Fats and Oils: The Complete Guide to Fats and Oils in Health and Nutrition.* Burnaby, British Columbia: Alive Books, 1991.

Hu, FB, et al. "Dietary intake of Alpha-Linolenic Acid and Risk of Fatal Ischemic Heart Disease Among Women." *American Journal of Clinical Nutrition,* 69(5): (1999).

Lowe, MR. "The effect of dieting on eating behaviors: A three-factor model." *Psychological Bulletin* (1993): 14.

Miller, JB, Wolever, TMS, Colacgiuri, S, Powell, KF. *The Glucose Revolution: The Authoritative Guide to the Glycemic Index.* New York, NY: Marlowe and Co., 1999.

Nestle, Marion. *Food Politics.* Berkeley, CA: University of California Press, 2002.

Pereira, MA, Karashov, AI, Evveling, CB, et al. "Fast-food habits, weight gain and insulin resistance (the CARDIA study): 15-year prospective analysis." *The Lancet* (January 2005): 1–7; 365(945S): 4–5.

Polivy, J, Herman, CP. "Dieting and bingeing: a causal analysis." *American Journal of Psychology* (1985): 40.

Revised International Table of Glycemic Index and Glycemic Load Values at www.ajcn.org/cgi/content/full/76/1/5#SEC2.

Rolls, BJ, Morris, E, Roe, LS. "Portion size of food affects energy intake in normal-weight and overweight men and women." *American Journal of Clinical Nutrition* (2002): 76.

Rolls, BJ. "The Supersizing of America: Portion Size and the Obesity Epidemic." *Nutrition Today* 38(2). (March 2003).

Sears, Barry. *Enter the Zone.* New York, NY: HarperCollins, 1995.

Steward, HL, Bethea, MC, Andrews, SS, Balart, LA. *Sugar Busters!* New York, NY: Ballantine Publishing Group, 1995.

Swain, A., Truswell, AS, Loblay, RH.. "Adverse reactions to food." *Food Technology in Australia* 36(10). (1984).

Vahouny, C., Kritchevsky, D. *Dietary Fiber in Health and Disease.* New York, NY: Plenum Press, 1982.

Wien, MA, Sabate, JM, Ikle, DN, et al. "Almonds vs. complex carbohydrates in a weight reduction program." *International Journal of Obesity* 27(11). (November 2003).

Wurtman, JJ, Zeisel, SH. "Carbohydrate craving in obese people." *International Journal of Eating Disorders,* Vol 1. (1982): 4.

Ziegler, PJ, Jonnalagadda, SS, Nelson, JA et al. "Contribution of meals and snacks to nutrient intake of male and female elite figure skaters during peak competitive season." *Journal of the American College of Nutrition* 21(2). (2003).

Index

About the Author

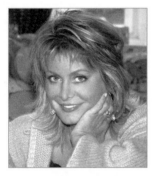

Deborah Arneson, B.S., M.S., L.C.N., is a licensed clinical nutritionist and an accredited member of the International Association of Clinical Nutritionists, the American Preventive Medical Association, the National Association of Ayurvedic Medicine, and the American Academy of Environmental Medicine.

In her more than two decades of experience, she has helped many people through counseling, consulting, speaking engagements, seminars, television appearances, and numerous magazine articles, all focused on the benefits of sound nutrition and healing. She practices at her Healing Quest Center in Chicago, Illinois, where she also lives.